OXFOR[illegible]

Breast Disease Management

Published and forthcoming Oxford Care Manuals

Stroke Care: A Practical Manual (2nd Edition)
Rowan Harwood, Farhad Huwez, and Dawn Good

Multiple Sclerosis Care: A Practical Manual
John Zajicek, Jennifer Freeman, and Bernadette Porter (eds)

Dementia Care: A Practical Manual
Jonathan Waite, Rowan H Harwood, Ian R Morton, and David J Connell

Headache: A Practical Manual
David Kernick and Peter J Goadsby (eds)

Diabetes Care: A Practical Manual
Rowan Hillson

Preventive Cardiology: A Practical Manual
Catriona Jennings, Alison Mead, Jennifer Jones, Annie Holden, Susan Connolly, Kornelia Kotseva, and David Wood

Neuromuscular Disorders in the Adult: A Practical Manual
David Hilton-Jones, Jane Freebody, and Jane Stein

Cardiovascular Disease in the Elderly: A Practical Manual
Rosaire Gray and Louise Pack

Motor Neuron Disease: A Practical Manual
Kevin Talbot, Martin R. Turner, Rachael Marsden, and Rachel Botell

Breast Disease Management: A Multidisciplinary Manual
James Harvey, Sue Down, Rachel Bright-Thomas, John Winstanley, and Hugh Bishop

Breast Disease Management

A Multidisciplinary Manual

James Harvey

Consultant Oncoplastic Breast Surgeon,
Nightingale Centre, UHSM, Manchester, UK

Sue Down

Consultant Oncoplastic Breast Surgeon, James Paget Hospital, UK; Hon. Senior Lecturer, University of East Anglia, UK

Rachel Bright-Thomas

Consultant Oncoplastic Breast Surgeon
Worcestershire Royal Hospital, UK

John Winstanley

Emeritus Consultant Surgeon, Royal Bolton Hospital, UK; Hon. Consultant Surgeon, Royal Liverpool and Broadgreen University Hospital, UK; Hon. Research Fellow, Biological Sciences, Liverpool University, UK

Hugh Bishop

Emeritus Consultant Surgeon, Royal Bolton Hospital, Bolton, UK

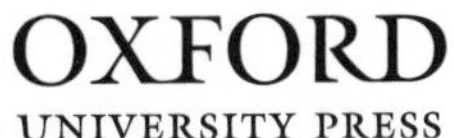
OXFORD
UNIVERSITY PRESS

OXFORD
UNIVERSITY PRESS

Great Clarendon Street, Oxford, OX2 6DP,
United Kingdom

Oxford University Press is a department of the University of Oxford. It furthers the University's objective of excellence in research, scholarship, and education by publishing worldwide. Oxford is a registered trade mark of Oxford University Press in the UK and in certain other countries

First Edition published in 2014

Impression: 1

Published in the United States of America by Oxford University Press
198 Madison Avenue, New York, NY 10016, United States of America

British Library Cataloguing in Publication Data
Data available

Library of Congress Control Number: 2013942099

ISBN 978–0–19–921506–5

Printed in Great Britain on acid-free paper by
Ashford Colour Press Ltd., Gosport, Hampshire.

Preface

As its name implies, this manual is intended to be of practical assistance to those working in the breast industry. Advances in breast cancer are such that it would be wrong for us to be dogmatic on fast-moving areas, such as molecular biology or chemotherapy. Nevertheless, the process of breast care has now evolved to be truly multidisciplinary.

This book is thus aimed at all members of the Multidisciplinary Team (MDT), however peripheral their contribution. We hope it will provide an introduction to all those medical professionals working in the field of breast disease, such as:

- Foundation doctors attached to breast firms.
- Core Trainees (CT 1&2) and Specialty Trainees (ST) with no prior knowledge or experience of breast firms.
- General practitioners with a breast interest.
- Specialist Breast Care Nurses.
- Medical students.
- Specialist breast radiographers.
- Breast physicians.
- Those who are responsible for purchasing or providing breast services.

In writing this book, we have concentrated on principles of care as they apply at present. We have deliberately avoided detailed information about:

- Advanced or rarely performed surgical operations.
- Chemotherapy regimens, as these change with each new publication or conference.
- Detailed issues of palliative care which are covered in 🕮 Oxford Handbook of Palliative Care, 2e (2009). Watson *et al.* Oxford University Press, Oxford, UK.

Whatever your discipline and whether or not you are embarking on a career in breast disease or merely transiting during your training, we hope you will find this book helpful in delivering excellent care to the patient with breast disease.

Hugh Bishop

Foreword

The past decade has seen some major advances in the management of breast disease. Better imaging and diagnostics, improved surgical and radiotherapy techniques together with more targeted drug therapies should lead to increased patient benefit. Good cooperation and communication within and between increasingly large multi-disciplinary teams is vital, as are management processes and systems that ensure the delivery of this improved care.

This is not always easy to achieve and can be a source of frustration to healthcare professionals and patients alike leading to sub-optimal care, complaints and litigation. Patients with benign breast disease, whilst spared the trauma provoked by a life-threatening diagnosis, nevertheless have problems that can be deeply distressing, embarrassing or painful. Some have signs and symptoms that create huge anxiety and considerable fears of a cancer diagnosis. Other patients may feel very well, will have no manifest breast lump or abnormalities, but may receive a sinister diagnosis following routine mammographic screening.

Whatever the aetiology and eventual diagnosis all patients need to be treated respectfully and sensitively by a multidisciplinary team contributing to management decisions from their own areas of expertise. This is only achievable with good teamwork, management experience and awareness of the important contributions that relevant disciplines might make to optimal decision-making.

The authors of this handbook have written a useful, pragmatic and broad introduction to the management of breast disease, taking account of some of the problems just mentioned and offering sensible, practical suggestions. The factual content is refreshingly succinct, with an occasional scintilla of humour and plenty of appropriate compassion. As such it avoids the rather prosaic, cold, and abstract feel of many such introductory manuals where one might just as well be reading about the maintenance of a piece of malfunctioning machinery rather than disease in a sensate being.

This text will be invaluable to anyone needing to acquire an overview or to begin work in this challenging but immensely rewarding clinical field.

Professor Lesley Fallowfield
Sussex Health Outcomes Research & Education in Cancer (SHORE-C),
Brighton & Sussex Medical School
University of Sussex, Falmer, UK
August 2013

Contents

Symbols and Abbreviations

°	degree
£	pound sterling
&	and
%	per cent
>	greater than
<	less than
=	equal to
±	with or without
~	approximately
π	pi
®	registered
™	trademark
ACE	angiotensin-converting enzyme
ADH	atypical ductal hyperplasia
ADRC	adipose-derived regenerative cell
A&E	Accident and Emergency
AI	aromatase inhibitor
AJCC	American Joint Committee on Cancer
ALH	atypical lobular hyperplasia
ANC	axillary node clearance
ANDI	aberrations of normal development and involution
BCN	breast care nurse
BCS	breast-conserving surgery
BMI	body mass index
CC	cranio-caudal
cm	centimetre
CT	Core Trainee
CVA	cerebrovascular accident
CXR	chest X-ray
DCIS	ductal carcinoma *in situ*
DEXA	dual-energy X-ray absorptiometry
DIEP	deep inferior epigastric perforators
DNA	deoxyribonucleic acid
DVT	deep vein thrombosis
EBCTCG	Early Breast Cancer Trials Collaborative Group

ECG	electrocardiogram
e.g.	*exempli gratia* (for example)
EGFR	epidermal growth factor receptor
ER	(o)estrogen receptor
ERP	Enhanced Recovery Programme
FBC	full blood count
FISH	fluorescent *in situ* hybridization
FNA	fine-needle aspiration
FNAC	fine-needle aspiration cytology
FRCS	Fellow of the Royal College of Surgeons
FY	Foundation Year
g	gram
GI	gastrointestinal
GP	general practitioner
GnRH	gonadotropin-releasing hormone
G&S	group and save
Gy	gray
h	hour
hCG	human chorionic gonadotropin
HRT	hormone replacement therapy
i.e.	*id est* (that is)
IHC	immunohistochemistry
IMF	inframammary fold
IT	information technology
IUCD	intrauterine contraceptive device
IV	intravenous
kg	kilogram
LCIS	lobular carcinoma *in situ*
LD	latissimus dorsi
LH	luteinizing hormone
LIN	lobular intraepithelial neoplasia
LREC	local research ethics committee
LVF	left ventricular function
m	metre
MDM	multidisciplinary meeting
MDT	multidisciplinary team
mg	milligram
mGy	milligray
mL	millilitre
MLO	mediolateral oblique

mm	millimetre
MREC	multicentre research ethics committee
MRI	magnetic resonance imaging
MRSA	Meticillin-resistant *Staphylococcus aureus*
MUGA	multigated acquisition (scan)
NAC	nipple-areola
NHS	National Health Service
NHSBSP	National Health Service Breast Screening Programme
NICE	National Institute for Health and Care Excellence
NMBRA	National Mastectomy and Breast Reconstruction Audit
NPI	Nottingham Prognostic Index
NST	no special type
OBCS	oncoplastic breast-conserving surgery
OCP	oral contraceptive pill
PCR	polymerase chain reaction
PE	pulmonary embolism
PRN	*pro re nata* (as needed)
QA	quality assurance
RCT	randomized controlled trial
ROLL	radioguided occult lesion localization
RR	relative risk
RT-PCR	reverse transcriptase-polymerase chain reaction
SIEP	superficial inferior epigastric perforators
SIGN	Scottish Intercollegiate Guidelines Network
SLN	sentinel lymph node
SLNB	sentinel lymph node biopsy
ST	Specialty Trainee
TB	tuberculosis
TDLU	terminal duct lobular unit
TED	thromboembolism deterrent
TNM	tumour, node, metastasis
TRAM	transverse rectus abdominis muscle
U&E	urea and electrolytes
UK	United Kingdom
U/S	ultrasound
US	United States
vs	versus
WBRT	whole breast radiotherapy
WHO	World Health Organization
WLE	wide local excision

[illegible]	[illegible]ampere
[illegible]	[illegible]
[illegible]	[illegible]
[illegible]	[illegible]
[illegible]	[illegible] (UK)
[illegible]	[illegible]
[illegible]	National Health Service
[illegible]	National Health Service Breast Screening Programme
[illegible]	National Institute for Health and Clinical Excellence
[illegible]	National Mastectomy and Breast Reconstruction Audit
[illegible]	Nottingham Prognostic Index
[illegible]	no special type
[illegible]	oncoplastic breast conserving surgery
[illegible]	[illegible]
[illegible]	polymerase chain reaction
[illegible]	progesterone receptor
[illegible]	pro re nata (as needed)
[illegible]	quality of life
[illegible]	randomized controlled trials
[illegible]	[illegible]
[illegible]	radiotherapy
[illegible]	[illegible]
[illegible]	superficial inferior epigastric perforator
[illegible]	Scottish Intercollegiate Guidelines Network
[illegible]	sentinel lymph node
[illegible]	sentinel lymph node biopsy
[illegible]	[illegible]
[illegible]	tamoxifen
[illegible]	terminal duct lobular unit
[illegible]	[illegible]
[illegible]	tumour, node, metastasis
[illegible]	transverse rectus abdominis myocutaneous flap
[illegible]	[illegible]
[illegible]	United Kingdom
[illegible]	ultrasound
[illegible]	United States
[illegible]	[illegible]
[illegible]	World Health Organization
[illegible]	wide local excision

Chapter 1

How to survive outpatient clinics in breast disease

Overview

Welcome to breast disease, one of the most fascinating areas of clinical medicine. To flourish in breast disease, it is vital to appreciate that it is a high-volume specialty. Unless you remain disciplined, your patients will suffer as a result of your inability to make a decision. Indecisiveness results in patients drifting into 'follow-up' clinics, often with disastrous results.

Success in breast disease depends on the successful working of a cohesive multidisciplinary team. This chapter looks at the patient's journey and where there is a potential danger to your patient.

Referral

It is normal to be worried, even frightened, by discovering a potential breast lump. Women naturally want the problem sorted and quickly. GPs are realistic and accept that, at the present time, a well-organized symptomatic breast clinic is the most efficient way to see, diagnose, and, more often than not, reassure and discharge the patient (hence, the huge number of referrals).

In addition, clinicians should be realistic. There is a political dimension to breast disease. All women have two breasts and one vote. This is reflected in the concern politicians demonstrate for breast cancer. There is a Breast Cancer Committee of the House of Commons. The Breast Cancer charities make a considerable contribution in terms of education, funding research as well as lobbying.

Breast clinicians wish to see and reassure patients as quickly as possible. To do this, it is not enough to examine a patient; breast patients require imaging. The problem arises because of insufficient numbers of breast radiologists. Not having a breast radiologist in the symptomatic clinic means patients may have to return two, or even three, times, which is upsetting to the patient as well as expensive and inefficient.

The referral letter

Beware that vital information on prescribed drugs or relevant history is often missing.

The symptomatic breast clinic

It is important to recognize that the ratio of new symptomatic breast patients to a patient with breast cancer is about 12–15:1. A great deal of the work of a symptomatic breast clinic is thus reassuring the worried well.

Most patients will require a clinical examination, breast imaging, reassurance, and, above all, discharge by the time the clinic has ended. Patients, when they make an appointment, should be advised that attendance at a breast clinic could take 3 hours.

Although some units are so pressed that patients are mammogrammed first, it is better to allow the patient to be seen clinically first. It is courteous to allow a patient to have an opportunity to explain their concerns. It also saves the time and trouble of performing mammography on a woman referred with a sebaceous cyst.

Furthermore, an initial history and examination allows the clinician to alert the breast radiologist to areas of clinical concern or problems, e.g. frozen shoulder. Most women in an NHS symptomatic breast clinic will end up with a double assessment, i.e. clinical assessment and breast imaging.

There is nothing to prevent a non-radiologist acquiring breast ultrasound (U/S) skills. There are courses and standards, but, at the present time, breast U/S is still the preserve of the breast radiologist. Since the best results are obtained when a biopsy is image-guided, then, in practice, it will be the radiologist who will perform the core biopsy.

The rate-limiting step in a contemporary NHS breast clinic is how fast the breast radiologist can comfortably work. This implies the clinician and the radiologist must agree what is possible to achieve in a session.

Most women in a symptomatic breast clinic will not have breast cancer, which means there will be no breast care nurses present—there are not enough of them anyway. This implies an adequate number of outpatient staff to assist in helping 20 women to undress, dress, go for imaging, undress, dress, wait, more imaging, undress, a needle biopsy, 5 minutes pressure on the needle site, and dress again before departure. Whilst some nurses will be required, a sensible lady with kindness and common sense can make the patient's experience much less distressing. We have been privileged to work with some outstanding Health Care Assistants with not a qualification to their name. Clinics should not habitually overrun, as this is unfair on patients and low-paid staff and is also inefficient, e.g. the last core biopsy specimen of the day goes missing because the laboratory has shut and the specimen was not properly signed in.

Managers may demand that patients are seen in order to meet a clinically irrelevant target. It is of no help to the patient if, because of a lack of a radiologist, the patient has to make two, or three, return visits in order to have her breast imaging and core biopsy. Worse still, a relatively unsupervised junior may then see the patient in a follow-up clinic. The cost of this muddled process far outweighs the cost of doing it right first time. Follow-up clinics containing patients with no clear diagnosis are a rich source of delay in diagnosis. For this reason, there must be good and documented reasons for a breast patient without breast cancer to require a return visit. In practice, most review appointments often involve a follow-up U/S, so arrange the appointment for when the patient, clinician, and radiologist are all present.

The distinguished psycho-oncologist Lesley Fallowfield has published evidence to suggest it is good practice for a patient without breast cancer to be seen, processed, and discharged in one session.

The same is not true of a woman who does have breast cancer and who will need adaptation time. The latter patient needs to leave the clinic with a time and date for her next appointment, together with the contact number for the breast care nurse. It is good practice for the clinician(s) and breast radiologist to go through the clinic list at the end of the clinic to ensure no obvious errors of omission have taken place.

Core biopsy

U/S-guided core biopsy is now the needling procedure of choice. Fine-needle aspiration cytology (FNAC) has effectively been abandoned for breast lesions and is best reserved for axillary node assessment.

The diagnostic multidisciplinary meeting (MDM)

All patients who have had a needling procedure require discussion at an MDM. The diagnostic MDM should recommend the range of surgical options that the patient can be offered. Patients should understand that a multidisciplinary discussion of their problem is required before an opinion can be given. It is poor practice to see a patient after a triple assessment if they have not been discussed in an MDM.

Post-MDM appointment

The breast care nurse should always be present when a patient receives the diagnosis of breast cancer. The patient needs time to come to terms with her options, particularly reconstructive options, and frequently needs more than one appointment before a decision is agreed.

Post-operative MDM

There is no point in discussing the patient, unless you have all the results. Patients must be alerted to this. The multidisciplinary team (MDT) should agree the adjuvant therapy programme to be offered. In addition, the follow-up schedule and mammographic surveillance programme must be agreed and documented. The intensity of follow-up will reflect the individual's inherent prognosis.

The post-operative consultation

Try to be truthful. Oncologists complain bitterly that, too often, surgeons avoid spelling out the true prognosis or need for treatment. The result is that the patient feels quite optimistic until the oncologist dashes this rosy outlook. The effect is to damage the oncologist/patient relationship and is devastating to the patient.

If necessary, make a list of the points you wish to convey, and remember to ensure the breast care nurse is with you.

Follow-up after breast cancer

Originally designed to detect recurrence, which nowadays follow-up clinics very seldom do. The emphasis has changed to encompassing issues of bone health, sexual health, and the side effects of adjuvant therapy.

Practically any symptom can be a potential manifestation of metastatic disease.

Assessing the post-operative, radiotherapized breast is not easy. Bear in mind that repeated requests for follow-up appointments may imply a need for psychological assistance.

In assessing symptomatic patients in a follow-up clinic, it is worth considering the patient's original prognostic factors, such as whether she was originally a symptomatic or screen-detected cancer, what her original NPI score and HER2 status were, and whether or not there was lymphovascular invasion.

Do not ignore life events, such as a husband's recent death or a daughter's divorce, which have been shown to be linked to the subsequent development of metastatic breast cancer. Sometimes, questioning may reveal the stress has been produced because a friend has developed recurrence or died, and this event has not unsurprisingly resurrected the patient's level of anxiety.

Oncoplastic surgery is technically challenging and is part of its appeal to surgical trainees. Nevertheless, there is much more to breast disease than complex operations. It is vital that the patient undergoes the most appropriate operation for her as an individual. Thus, the process of consenting is an important aspect of outpatient work. In addition, the considerable diagnostic load has to be handled accurately and sensitively. Finally, follow-up and mammographic surveillance need to be set out for the patient on an individual basis.

Welcome to breast disease.

Chapter 2

The National Health Service Breast Screening Programme (NHSBSP)

History

The decision to fund an NHSBSP was taken following a report by Professor Sir Patrick Forrest and is known as the Forrest Report. Forrest reviewed all the evidence at that time, 1986, and concluded that mammographic screening had the potential to reduce mortality from breast cancer in the UK population. The greatest benefit was in older women. It was not considered that younger women would derive any benefit. For this reason, the NHSBSP set out to screen all women who were aged between 50 and 65.

Principles of screening

The general principles of screening for any disease are that:

- The disease screened for represents an important health problem.
- It has a well-understood natural history.
- It has a recognizable early stage.
- There is a benefit from early treatment.
- There is a suitable test.
- It is acceptable to the population.
- There are adequate facilities to diagnose and treat the condition.
- Screening can be done at intervals to match the natural history.
- There is less harm than benefit.

Two measures are considered in this, which apply to any test—these are the sensitivity and the specificity.

The sensitivity of a test is a measure of its ability to identify true positive cases. The specificity is the ability to identify true negative cases (see Table 2.1).

Sensitivity = a/a + b
Specificity = d/c + d

Expressed as percentages, an ideal test has a high percentage for both sensitivity and specificity. In breast cancer terms, the purpose of the screening programme is not to diagnose cancers but to reduce mortality from breast cancer in the population.

Statistics

At the present time, the screening programme screens 1.88 million women a year and diagnoses 14,725 breast cancers per year (2010–11) (see Further reading).

This work is carried out by:

- 80 breast screening units.
- Cost—£96 million/year.
- 73.4% of those invited for screening attend for their screen.
- 79.5% invasive cancers vs 20.5% DCIS.
- Rate of recall for further assessment—40 per 1,000 women screened.
- Rate of biopsy of the breast following further assessment—17 per 1,000 women screened.
- Rate of cancer detection is 7.8 cases per 1,000 women screened.

Table 2.1 Definition of the sensitivity and the specificity of a test

	Patient with breast cancer	**Patient without breast cancer**
Test positive for breast cancer	True positive (a)	False positive (c)
Test negative for breast cancer	False negative (b)	True negative (d)

Organization of breast screening

Forrest proposed that a breast screening unit should serve a catchment population of 500,000. Broadly, this 'Forrest unit' structure has persisted, although there are now some very large units. The NHSBSP built on lessons learnt from earlier screening programmes. The most important was an emphasis on quality assurance (QA—a new concept to many surgeons in 1988!). Subsequently, the NHSBSP has developed a robust audit structure in order to improve the service. A senior NHS manager heads the programme, and regional screening teams are assisted by regional QA committees, consisting of all the disciplines participating in the programme (see Fig. 2.1).

It is important to understand that the screening service is organizationally separate from a hospital breast unit. In many instances, it will be based in a particular hospital's breast unit so that, to all intents and purposes, it will appear as one unit, but it will have a clerical staff that is separate from the hospital's clerical staff; in some instances, the radiographers will be separate, and some of the radiologists may not do routine screening film reading. Because of the large geographical areas involved, there will be, in addition to a static screening unit, several mobile units, all administered by the central unit. For that reason, not every hospital that treats breast cancer is a screening unit. From a technical point of view, women undergoing screening are not called patients but clients. They only become patients when they have either a cancer diagnosed or some other abnormality requiring surgical intervention, commonly a core biopsy. At that point, they become a patient and are referred to a surgeon. In many instances, that will be an in-house referral to a surgeon working in the breast unit of which the screening unit is a part. However, given the large areas covered by screening units, it might be more convenient for patients to be treated at a hospital more local to them, in which case a screening unit must have an arrangement to repatriate local patients to a particular hospital. Nevertheless, the hospital must demonstrate that its surgeons and radiologists have the knowledge and facilities to carry out such procedures as wire-guided biopsies, local excisions, and sentinel node biopsies. At present, there is a distinction made between symptomatic and screening breast units. It is recognized that the skills acquired in breast screening, particularly in radiology, are of major benefit in symptomatic practice. There is, therefore, a move to try to integrate the two services. Those hospitals that do not have a screening programme must work to the same standards of diagnostic stringency that screening units are required to demonstrate.

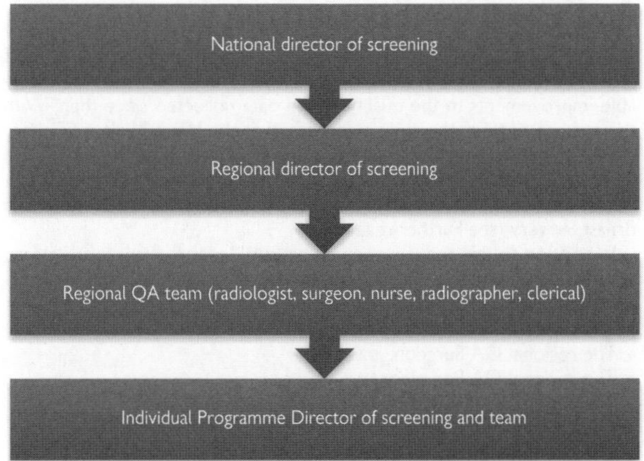

Fig. 2.1 The organizational structure of the NHSBSP.

Audit and quality control

The NHSBSP audit of screen-detected breast cancer made its first attempt at collecting screening data in 1996. There have been considerable improvements in the quality of the data collected since then. With the passage of time, the audit team, based at the West Midlands Cancer Intelligence Unit, have been able to report 5-year survival rates and, quite recently, 20-year survival rates for screen-detected cancers. The audit results are presented annually at the annual meeting of the Association of Breast Surgery (see Further reading).

In addition to this annual review at national level, there is local review, which takes place every 3 years. This is done by the regional quality assurance team. This consists of:

- The regional Director of Screening.
- The regional QA Surgeon.
- The regional QA Radiologist.
- The regional QA Pathologist.
- The regional QA Radiographer.
- The regional QA Breast Care Nurse.
- The regional QA Clerical Officer.
- The regional QA Physicist.

This team visits each of the screening units within the region once every 3 years and audits their performance against the screening guidelines; this includes an assessment of the operation of the radiology equipment. The purpose is to praise good practice and offer suggestions where they feel performance could be enhanced. Many teams find the visits can be helpful. External support for improvements in a written report is less easy for managers to ignore!

National screening committees for each discipline–the BIG 18s

Each of the clinical disciplines—surgery, radiology, pathology, breast care nurses, and radiographers—has a national committee, of which the regional QA representative is a member. These became known as the BIG 18s because there were originally 18 screening regions. The national committees meet twice a year. Their function is to discuss issues affecting the screening programmes and formulate policy. These groups oversee revision of the various guidelines for the disciplines, which is conducted on a regular basis. For example, the national committee for pathology in breast screening recently made a formal recommendation that core biopsy was the needling procedure of choice in screen-detected lesions and that, within the NHSBSP, fine-needle aspiration cytology should be abandoned.

The screening process

At the start of the programme, screening was targeted at the 50–65 year old age group. However, this was extended to take the age limit up to 70, and the plan in the future is to extend the programme to include all women from 47–73.

Women are screened by general practice lists once every 3 years. A common misconception is that once a woman becomes 50, she will be called for screening. This is not the case; she will only be called when her practice is screened. For example, if a lady turns 50 six months after her practice was screened, she will not be screened until the practice is next screened in 3 years. The process is summarized in Fig. 2.2. After the upper age limit of routine invitation for screening, a woman remains eligible for screening every 3 years, however, the request has to be made by the individual patient to the local screening unit.

- Patients are invited to be screened as a group from a general practice triennially. The first invitation occurs between 50 and 53 years of age. Any client who has had mammography within the previous 12 months is advised not to undergo screening in this round.
- Two view (cranio-caudal and lateral-oblique) screening mammograms are taken of each breast in a static or mobile screening unit. A patient questionnaire is also completed, giving basic relevant history, which is available to the mammogram readers.
- The majority of clients are returned to 'routine recall' in 3 years' time—written confirmation is sent to the client.
- Those with a possible abnormality on their screening mammograms (such as micro-calcification, mass, asymmetric density, distortion) or those who have mentioned a significant new clinical problem on their questionnaire are recalled to an assessment clinic.

The assessment procedure

This can involve the following stages:

- Further mammographic views—repeat standard views, coned compression views, magnification views.
- Clinical examination.
- Ultrasound scanning.

If a radiological or clinical abnormality persists, a needle biopsy is undertaken.

- Ultrasound-guided biopsies. Possible for focal abnormalities visible on ultrasound, e.g. mass or distortion and sometimes for micro-calcification.
- Mammographic, stereotactically guided biopsies. Done for micro-calcification or for lesions not visible on ultrasound.
- Clinically guided biopsies can be undertaken for palpable lesions.
- Specimens are radiographed to check for the presence of micro-calcification.

Biopsy procedures

All are done under local anaesthetic.

The multidisciplinary team meeting (MDT)

This has been another of the big benefits conferred on cancer management in general from the breast screening process. It is a requirement of

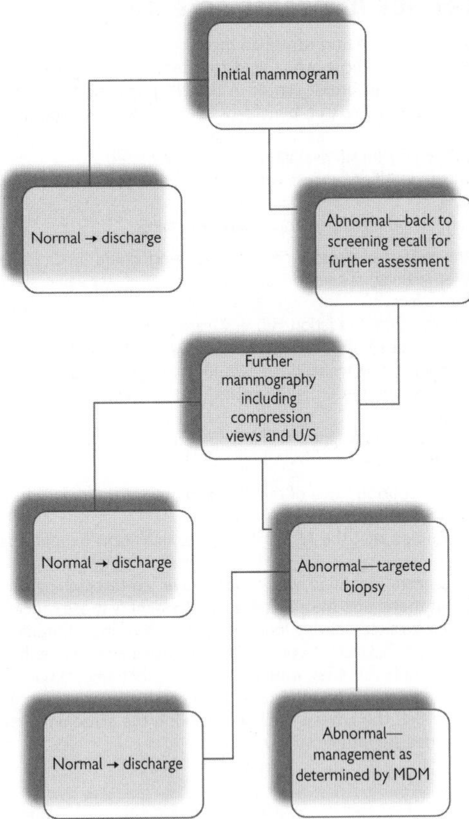

Fig. 2.2 Flow of patients through the breast screening process to diagnosis.

the QA process that units have a regular meeting to discuss the results of patients who are of concern. This usually comprises:

- Patients who have undergone biopsy.
- Patients whose mammograms require group discussion.

This meeting allows a group decision on how best to manage the problem identified. This usually results in a consistent standard of treatment and avoids patients being subjected to idiosyncratic variability. As part of the QA process, a representative of the QA usually attends one meeting, unannounced, to write a report on the conduct of the meeting. As with other MDT meetings, the proceedings must be recorded and a register kept.

Controversies in breast screening

The 20-year survival data demonstrate an increase in survival in women screened compared with those who failed to attend. The original remit was to reduce death from breast cancer in the UK population. There is some controversy about the true benefit of breast screening. The main areas of concern are:

- The statistical benefit on survival has been overestimated.
- The programme identifies cancers which would never be life-threatening.
- The process of screening is psychologically disturbing.

An independent review of breast screening was performed in October 2012 (see Further reading). Their conclusions, based on a meta-analysis of the available data, were:

- NHSBSP leads to a 20% reduction in breast cancer mortality.
- One breast cancer death is prevented for every 250 women invited.
- 19% of cancers are overdiagnosed (i.e. would not have caused harm to the patient if left alone) during the period that women are in the screening programme.
- 11% of all breast cancers diagnosed in a woman's lifetime constitute overdiagnosis.

These figures give a spurious idea of the true accuracy of the data, which have a large confidence interval.

The panel concluded that the NHSBSP confers significant benefit and should continue.

Some of the cancers identified would not prove life-threatening, the problem being that there is no means, at present, to identify those cancers so that not treating a cancer, having found it, would be taking a considerable gamble. It is true that some women find the process worrying, but, on balance, most people feel they would rather have that anxiety and be diagnosed early rather than allow the tumour to reach a more advanced stage. It is unlikely that the government will abandon the screening programme in the immediate future.

Future developments

- Digital mammographic screening for all screening units.
- An age extension trial is currently underway of women aged 47–50 and 70–73 to determine whether screening is of benefit.
- Developing an audit of screen-detected non-invasive breast cancer. This audit, called the Sloane Project, is now complete (see Further reading), and over 11,000 women have been enrolled (November 2012). This is the largest prospective audit of non-invasive screen-detected breast cancer to date.

Further reading

Further information on breast screening, including statistical data, can be found at: http://www.cancerscreening.nhs.uk/breastscreen/index.html

Independent review on breast cancer screening. Available at: http://www.cancerresearchuk.org

Sloane project. Available at: http://www.sloaneproject.co.uk

Chapter 3

Multidisciplinary working

Overview

Patients with breast symptoms are managed by a multidisciplinary team for their diagnosis and at all stages of their treatment. This implies mutual respect for the various disciplines involved in the process.

The multidisciplinary team (MDT)

Composition of the MDT

[illegible]

Functions of the MDT

[illegible]

The multidisciplinary team (MDT)

Components of the MDT

A modern breast MDT needs the following components:
- Surgeons.
- Radiologists.
- Pathologists.
- Oncologists.
- Breast care nurses.
- An MDT coordinator and adequate clerical support.
- Data manager.
- Trials nurses.

These are the fundamental components, however, it is important that the team has links with other groups:-
- Plastics surgeons.
- Psychologists.
- Clinical geneticists.

It is important that the team has formally established mechanisms for referral to groups, such as oncologists, or other centres that regularly form part of the patient journey. It is also important to have a good clerical and administrative infrastructure to ensure that all parts of the process happen. It is no use making good clinical decisions if clinic appointments are not booked or the GP does not get letters! Equally, team meetings need administrative support to ensure that all the films, notes, and pathology reports are assembled together. There are now systems in place to record the data and decisions made in real time online, e.g. Somerset Health Informatics Database. The results are immediately available to team members. It is wrong to discuss results if one component (e.g. Her-2 result) is missing. Failure to have all results present or to have representation from each of the fundamental disciplines can result in catastrophic failure.

Functions of the MDT

The MDT has a number of functions:
- To plan and organize treatment for both benign and malignant breast disease.
- To establish a cycle of audit and research.
- To act as a focus for undergraduate and postgraduate education in breast diseases.
- To advise local healthcare providers on provision of services.
- To establish a trials portfolio.
- To determine operational policies and protocols.

How individual teams organize themselves is, in part, controlled by local circumstances, but, in order to function well, all teams need:
- Operational policies so that everyone knows how to handle specific situations.
- Regular meetings so that all patients undergoing diagnostic procedures and surgery are discussed.

- Regular meetings to discuss the way the unit functions on a day-to-day basis, to review protocols as well as discuss complaints and errors.
- A written record of all decisions made by the MDT.
- An easily accessible database.
- Time to carry out all this.
- An MDM should be part of an individual's job plan.

Most units will have a lead clinician. But if a team is going to function well, it is vital that everyone involved feels valued for the contribution they make, and that is why regular meetings are important to allow all those involved to express their views, be it on clinical or organizational matters. When this does not happen, teams become dysfunctional and break down, which ultimately leads to clinical errors.

Much of modern breast management is about process, and it is important for the team that the process is recorded both clinically and from a medico-legal point of view. Notes can get lost, and a record of what happened in the meeting held separately is supportive.

It is important that timetabling is such that all members can get to meetings; if the oncologist cannot get to the meetings, they cease to be multidisciplinary. It is also important that adequate time is allowed; fitting meetings in between sandwiches at lunch time is often another recipe for disaster in a busy unit.

Apart from clinical meetings, it is important that teams meet regularly to look at operational matters. Working practices change, and what would have been appropriate 2 years previously may not be now. Similarly, changes in referral pattern may demand some re-organization of clinics. Responses made on the spur of the moment often end up needing to be revised. Equally important is audit and research (see Chapter 25). Audit is a requirement of modern practice. It also provides a focus of interest and avoids the danger of work becoming routine and the team becoming bored. In addition, it is a means of making sure that the team is functioning efficiently, which ultimately is in the best interests of patients.

Team communication

It is vital that team members, particularly those involved in clinical decisions, make their opinions clear to their colleagues. Many clinical problems arise because of a breakdown in this aspect of multidisciplinary working. Those examining patients need to make their opinion clear about whether lesions are sinister or not and if further imaging is needed should the mammogram appear normal. Similarly, radiologists and pathologists need to give a clear indication of their views on the nature of a lesion so that all those involved have clear opinions to base their decisions on.

Conclusion

Multidisciplinary working is now established as an important component of managing patients with breast problems. A functional MDT will have patients who feel that their management is in safe hands, receiving consistent explanations of their treatment, and the sense that the team knows what is going on. This can only be achieved if everyone works as a team member and not as an individual. Finally, good multidisciplinary working results in fewer mistakes.

Chapter 4

Anatomy and physiology

The breast

Embryology and developmental variants

Breasts are modified sweat glands, developing from ventral mammary ridges (the milk line) that run from the axilla to the inguinal region. Two common problems are (see Chapter 7):

- Accessory nipples and breasts: remnants of the embryonic tissue can remain anywhere along the milk line and be seen in adulthood as accessory breasts (usually as a bulge in the axilla) or as nipples just below the normal breast.
- Poland's syndrome: covers a wide variety of developmental failures of the chest wall and breasts, ranging from mild hypoplasia and asymmetry of the breast to complete absence of the breast and pectoral muscles with deformities of the rib cage and upper limb.

Anatomy

The huge variation in shape and size of the breast is related to the deposition of fat and stroma, but the anatomical landmarks are constant despite the variation in size and shape of the breast.

Breasts are never completely symmetrical. The left breast is commonly larger and more ptotic by a centimetre or two. The lack of symmetry can be highlighted by chest wall asymmetry. In general, breasts share these common features (see Figs 4.1 and 4.2):

- Modified sweat gland, comma-shaped with the tail extending towards the axilla.
- The breast base lies on pectoralis major, serratus anterior, rectus sheath.
- Overlies 2nd–6th ribs.
- Enveloped by the superficial fascia (Scarpas).
- Fibrous suspensory ligaments run through the breast, connecting skin to the deep layer of the superficial fascia (Cooper's ligaments).
- Rich lymphatic plexus (deep and superficial).
- Preferential lymphatic drainage toward the axilla (80%).

Structure

The adult female breast comprises both fatty and glandular tissue (see Fig. 4.3).

- Lobes 15–20. Each lobe is made up of many lobules, at the end of which are tiny bulb-like glands where milk is produced in response to hormonal signals—the terminal duct lobular unit (TDLU).
- The male breast does not contain TDLU. The TDLU are the functional part of the breast, and this is where most benign and malignant pathology arises.
- Duct system. The ducts connect the lobes to the lactiferous sinuses beneath the areola and 15–20 ducts ending on the nipple where the epithelium of the duct changes to squamous epithelium.
- Nipple-areola complex (NAC): The nipple and areola contain smooth muscle and modified sebaceous glands.

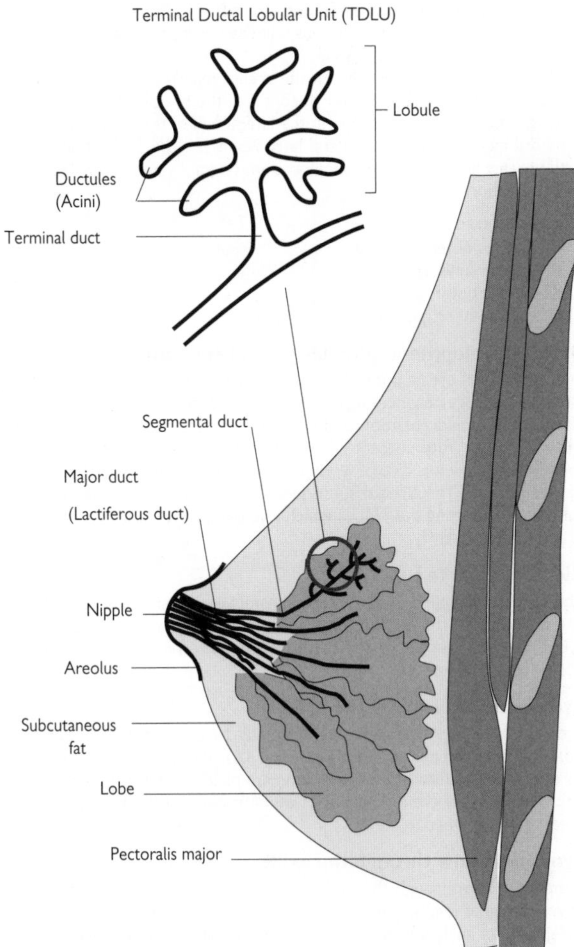

Fig. 4.1 Cross-section of the female breast. Reproduced with permission from 'Training in Surgery : The essential curriculum for the MRCS', edited by Matthew Gardiner, Neil Borley, copyright 2009 Oxford University Press.

It is supported and encased by fat and stroma.

- The stroma and fat (subcutaneous adipose tissue) that cover the lobes give the breast its size and shape.
- TDLUs lie scattered throughout the breast, mainly in the lateral half and especially the upper outer quadrant of the breast. This is why most breast pathology occurs in the lateral half of the breast. The medial half is mainly stromal and fatty tissue. It is the TDLU that gives the breast its dense appearance on mammography and lumpy feeling on palpation.

Site of cancers

- 50%: upper outer quadrant.
- 20%: upper inner quadrant.
- 20% lower outer quadrant.
- 10% lower inner quadrant.

Breast development, physiology, and endocrinology

Initial growth of breast buds occurs at puberty under the influence of oestrogen and progesterone. Oestrogen induces duct sprouting, and progesterone causes differentiation of the terminal lobular ducts to form lobules and the TDLU. Fifty percent of women have a 10% difference between their breast volumes, 25% of women have a 25% difference in the volume of their breasts. Throughout subsequent menstrual cycles, there are cyclical changes affecting the TDLU, which give rise to cyclical symptoms, such as pain and nodularity.

Blood and nerve supply

The breast is supplied by the internal mammary, anterior intercostal, and lateral thoracic arteries and their accompanying veins (see Figs 4.2 and 4.4). The nerve supply to the breast is primarily via intercostal sensory fibres (see Fig. 4.5).

Lymphatic drainage of the breast

Breast tissue lymphatics drain centripetally to a subareolar plexus and, from there, to the axillary nodes (see Fig. 4.6). Some of the deeper breast parenchyma also flows to a retromammary plexus and, from there, to the internal mammary chain. There are lymphatic connections to the opposite breast and abdomen.

Lymphatic flow through the axilla

Lymphatic flow through the axilla is orderly and tends to flow from the lower to higher levels, eventually draining into the neck. However, different groups of axillary nodes will preferentially drain different areas of the breast, arm, and chest. However, there is huge variability, especially in the presence of malignant nodal disease, which may obstruct, and so alter lymphatic flow and drainage patterns.

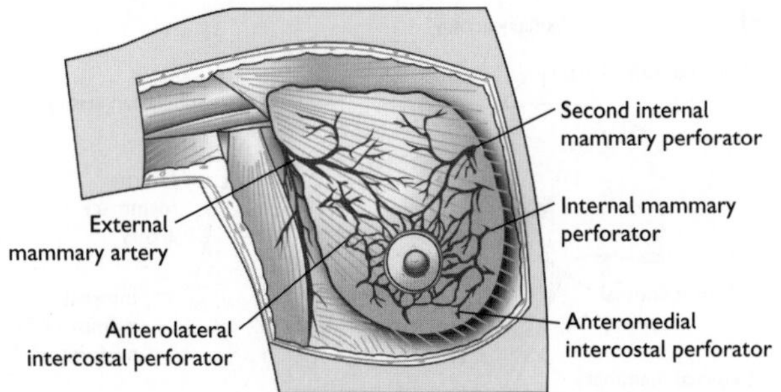

Fig. 4.2 Surface anatomy and blood supply of the breast. The breast overlies the 2nd–6th ribs, pectoralis major superiorly, and serratus anterior inferiorly. The blood supply is from branches of the lateral thoracic (external mammary), internal thoracic, and intercostal perforator arteries.

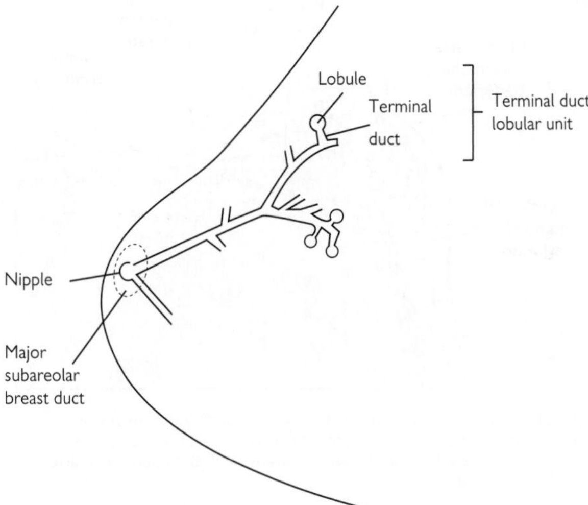

Fig. 4.3 Structure of breast tissue. The terminal duct lobular units are glands that open into the ducts of the breast, running towards the nipple. The ducts open into lactiferous sinuses behind the nipple before exiting via 15–20 ducts onto the nipple surface.

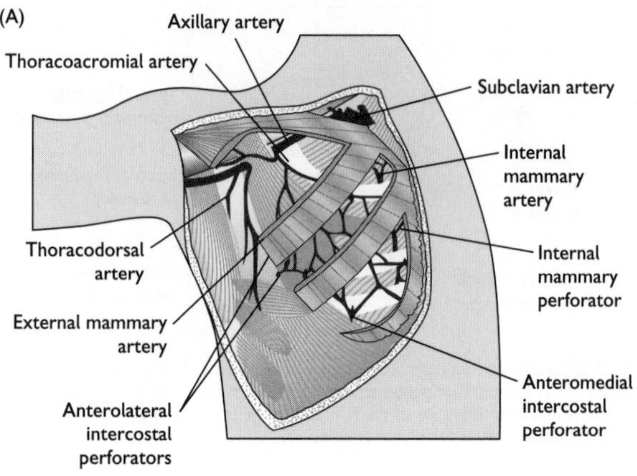

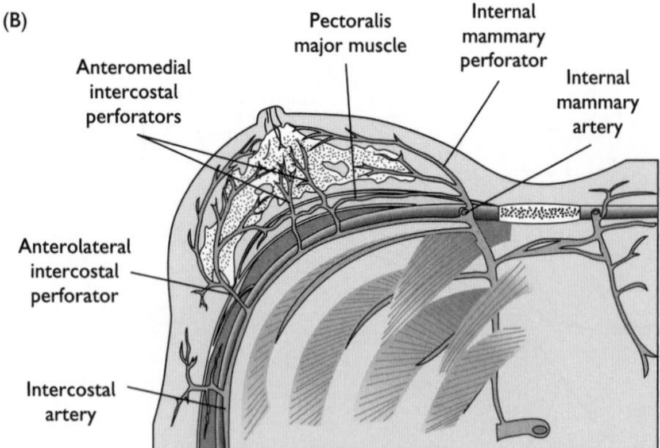

Fig. 4.4 Frontal view (A) and transverse view (B) of the right breast from below, demonstrating the blood supply of the breast. The breast is supplied by (A) branches of the subclavian and axillary arteries and (B) by perforating arteries from the intercostal vessels.

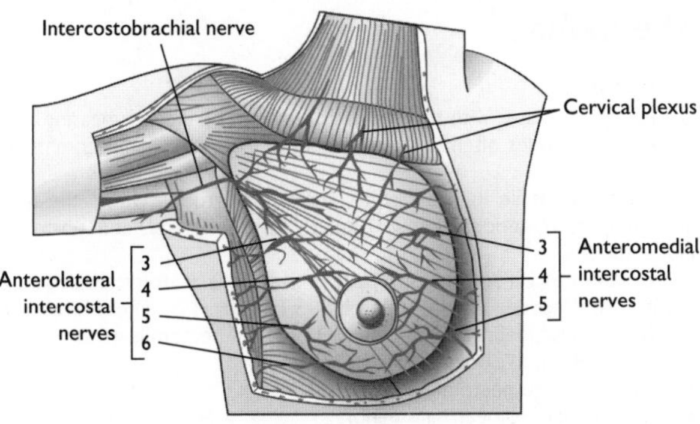

Fig. 4.5 Nerve supply of the breast. Primarily, branches of the intercostal nerves supply the breast; some additional sensation is supplied via the lower branches of the cervical plexus.

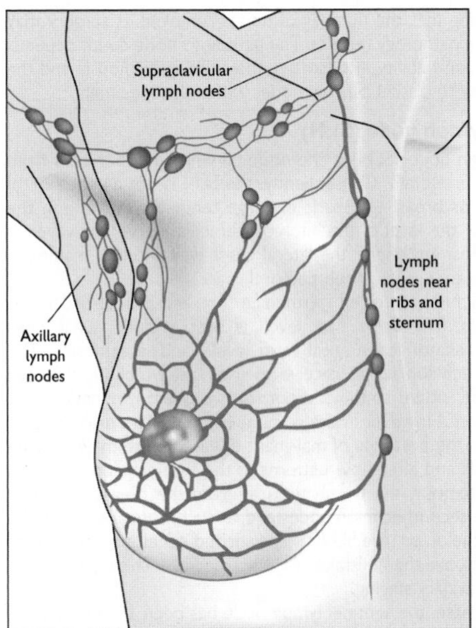

Fig. 4.6 Lymphatic drainage of the breast. The majority of the breast drains via the subareolar plexus to the axillary nodes. Medial areas can preferentially drain to the internal mammary chain.

The axilla

Anatomy

Is a pyramidal shape, with the base being formed by the hair-bearing area of axilla. The nodes often lie much deeper in the axilla than is commonly appreciated.

Axillary nodes lie in five distinct anatomical groups within the axillary fat/space: anterior (pectoral) apical, central, lateral, and posterior (subscapular).

From the surgical or functional perspective, these anatomically separate groups are described as lying in levels 1–3 (see Fig. 4.7). These levels run caudal to cranial, defined by the lateral border of pectoralis minor.

- Level 1: lateral to pectoralis minor.
- Level 2: deep to pectoralis minor.
- Level 3: medial to pectoralis minor.

The number of axillary nodes is variable, depending on body habitus. The central, anterior, and posterior groups account for the vast majority of nodes. As the level of dissection increases, the number of nodes harvested decreases: level 1 may contain approximately 10–15 nodes, with only 3 or 4 found in level 3.

It is worth noting that the number of nodes removed at surgery may not be reflected in pathology reports. The pathology node count depends on both the surgeon's ability in dissecting the axilla meticulously and the pathologist's ability to dissect out the nodes within the specimen.

The sentinel lymph node (SLN)

The sentinel lymph node (SLN) is the node to which tumour cells from a primary cancer first drain. Consequently, the SLN is not an anatomical entity. The SLN for breast lymphatic drainage tends to (80%) lie in the lower axilla below the level of the intercostobrachial nerve. However, it can be found almost anywhere: the lateral chest wall, internal mammary chain, intra-mammary tissue, or sub-pectoral space.

The axillary SLN(s) is often termed a first-level, first-order, or first-echelon node. The term 'first level' is best avoided, as it does not relate to the anatomical/surgical term level I and is confusing. The second-order or echelon nodes receive their breast lymphatic drainage from the first-order nodes so they do not receive direct lymphatic drainage from the cancer. However, there is variability in axillary drainage patterns, especially in the presence of malignant disease, which may obstruct lymphatic channels and alter flow patterns. If the first-echelon SLN(s) is obstructed with tumour, the lymphatic flow from the breast may then drain towards the second-echelon nodes and, as such, appear to 'skip' the cancerous first-echelon or true SLN(s). The second-echelon nodes, which may be cancer-free, are then mistaken for the true SLN. This may result in a falsely negative axillary staging.

In malignant disease, the sentinel lymph node has been shown to accurately predict the nodal status of the rest of the nodal basin. For example, if the axillary SLN is cancer-free, the rest of the axillary nodes will be cancer-free. If the SLN contains cancer, there is a 50% likelihood of further cancer in other axillary nodes.

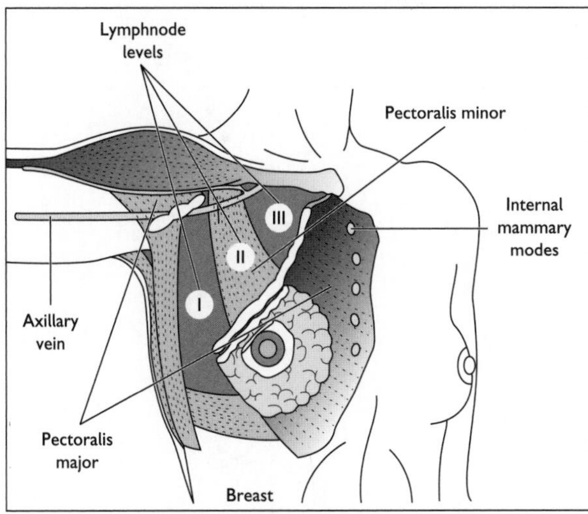

Fig. 4.7 Levels of the axillary lymph nodes. Axillary lymph nodes lie lateral to pectoralis minor (level I), deep to the muscle belly (level II), or medial to the muscle (level III). Reproduced with permission from Chaudry MA and Winslet MC, 'The Oxford Specialist Handbook of Surgical Oncology', copyright 2009, Oxford University Press.

Chapter 5

Breast cancer—facts and figures

Epidemiology

Incidence and geographic variation

According to the WHO, more than 1.2 million women worldwide are diagnosed with breast cancer each year, making it responsible for 22% of female cancers and 10% of all cancers. Incidence rates are greatest in the developed world but vary, even within Europe (see Fig. 5.1). Interestingly, migrants acquire the risk of their host country within two generations.

In Britain, the incidence of breast cancer has increased by 46% over the last 20 years. This is mirrored by a similar rise internationally (0.5% annually), but it is rising particularly fast in China and Eastern Asia (3–4% annually) where, historically, the incidence has been low. If non-melanoma skin cancer is excluded, breast cancer is now the most common cancer diagnosed in the UK (over 40,000 new cases in 2000), with over 100 new diagnoses each day.

Prevalence

Given the high incidence and good survival, the prevalence is high, with over 172,000 women in the UK having had a diagnosis of breast cancer.

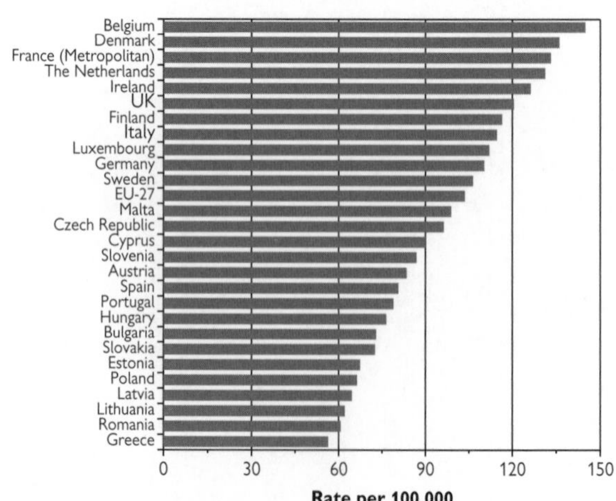

Fig. 5.1 European age-standardized incidence rates of breast cancer. Figure courtesy of Cancer Research UK EU 27 countries, 2008. Accessed Sept 2012. http://info.cancerresearchuk.org/cancerstats/types/breast/incidence/uk-breast-cancer-incidence-statistics#world

Survival

Survival is intimately linked to stage at diagnosis, but overall breast cancer-specific survival rates have steadily improved over the last 30 years (see Fig. 5.2).

- The 5-year survival rate for all women diagnosed with breast cancer in England and Wales is now >77%.
- Considering only screen-detected breast cancers, this rises to >95% because screen-detected cancers have a better survival outcome than symptomatic cancers, even when adjusted for tumour stage (see Further reading).

These good survival figures are likely to be due to a combination of factors, including uptake of breast screening, increasing specialization of care, and the use of tamoxifen and chemotherapy.

Survival is also affected by socio-economic status, with a statistically significant deprivation gap of >5% in 5-year survival between the top and bottom groups. This appears to be due to greater co-morbidity in socially deprived individuals rather than a difference in the standard of care.

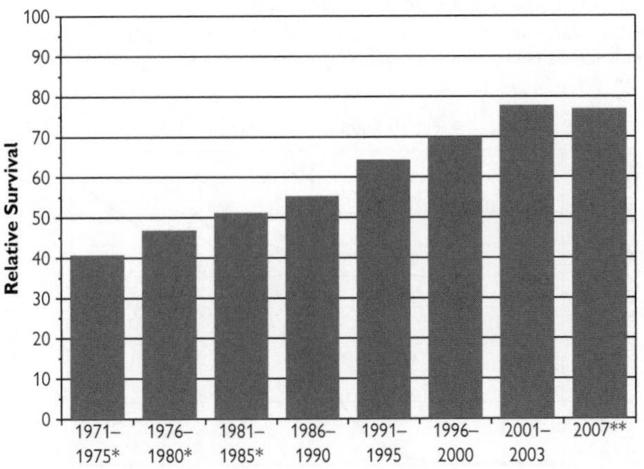

Fig. 5.2 Age-standardized 10-year relative survival rates, females, England and Wales 1971–1995 and predicted 2007, England 1996–2003. Figure courtesy of Cancer Research. Accessed Sept 2012. http://info.cancerresearchuk.org/cancerstats/types/breast/survival/

Risk factors for developing breast cancer

The four main risk factors are gender, age, a previous history of breast cancer, or a significant family history. Then, there are a host of lower risk factors which can be assessed. These will be discussed briefly.

Gender

Ninety-nine percent of cases are in women, in whom the lifetime risk is 1 in 9. However, men are not immune, and there are approximately 250 new cases of male breast cancer in the UK each year.

Age

Over 80% of cases occur in women over 50 years of age. It is rare under 30 but is the commonest cancer diagnosed in women under 35. The greatest rate of rise in incidence is just prior to the menopause, reflecting a hormonal association (see Fig. 5.3).

Previous history of breast cancer

Having had a previous breast cancer, the chance of developing a second breast primary is two to six times that of the general population risk of developing a first breast cancer.

Family history/genetic predisposition

Having one affected first-degree relative (mother or sister) doubles an individual's background risk of breast cancer, and a stronger family history

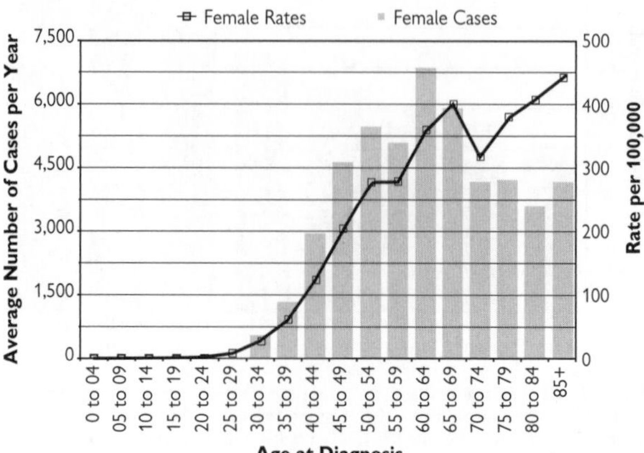

Fig. 5.3 Average number of new cases per year and age-specific incidence rates in females in the UK, 2008–2010. Figure courtesy of Cancer Research UK. Accessed Sept 2012. http://info.cancerresearchuk.org/cancerstats/types/breast/incidence/#age

increases risk still further. Women likely to be at increased risk of breast cancer should have their family history assessed to see if they would benefit from additional breast screening, possibly with genetic testing (see Further reading for NICE family history guidance and Chapter 24).

Reproductive/hormonal factors

The greater the period of unopposed oestrogen exposure (or number of menstrual cycles), the higher the risk of breast cancer. However, individually, these give small increases in relative risk rather than any individual factor being of great importance in its own right. Thus, risk is increased by:

- Lower age at menarche.
- Greater age at menopause.
- Greater age at first child.
- Nulliparity.
- Absence of, or reduced, period spent breastfeeding.
- Use of the oral contraceptive pill. Relative risk (RR) is increased to 1.24 during the period of use. Individual risk returns to baseline by 10 years after stopping.
- Use of hormone replacement therapy (HRT). The 'Million Women' study in 2003 showed an RR of 1.66 of developing breast cancer if a current user of HRT (see Further reading). However, the risk fell off dramatically in past users (1.01). When looking specifically at different types of HRT, it was highest for combined HRT (2.00) but was still increased with oestrogen-only compounds (1.3) and tibolone (1.45). Given these risks and the recent demonstration that HRT is also linked with an excess of stroke and venous thromboembolism, it is no longer recommended as a prophylactic measure to prevent osteoporosis or cardiovascular disease in all menopausal women. HRT should be reserved as a treatment for those women whose quality of life is affected by menopausal symptoms. Here, the risks and benefits can be assessed on an individual basis.

Physical factors

- Post-menopausal obesity. Adipose tissue is a source of extra-gonadal oestrogen production. Thus, there is an RR of 1.3 for a body mass index (BMI) of $>28\text{kg/m}^2$ compared with a BMI of $<20\text{kg/m}^2$). Premenopausal obesity does not have the same effect, possibly because it is often linked to an increased number of anovulatory cycles.
- Height. Taller women have an increased risk; the reason is unclear.

Lifestyle factors

- Diet. High levels of saturated animal fats may slightly increase risk.
- Alcohol. There is an association between alcohol intake and breast cancer.
- Physical activity. A few hours of vigorous exercise per week reduces risk (RR 0.7). It is unclear whether this is related to a drop in BMI or a direct alteration in hormonal levels.
- Socio-economic status is directly related to breast cancer incidence. This may simply reflect better early nutrition and delayed childbearing in the upper socio-economic groups.

Table 5.1 Risk of subsequent breast cancer associated with benign breast disease

Benign change	Relative risk of later breast cancer
Proliferative breast change (florid, usual-type hyperplasia), sclerosing adenosis, multiple papillomas	1.5x
Atypical ductal hyperplasia	4x
Lobular carcinoma *in situ*	10x

Breast factors

- Mammographic density. Denser breasts are associated with an increased risk of breast cancer (2–6-fold) and are harder to screen mammographically.
- Benign breast change. Some benign breast conditions are associated with an increased risk of subsequent breast cancer (see Table 5.1).
- Previous ionizing radiation to the chest. Clinically important in women previously treated for Hodgkin's lymphoma with mantle irradiation. One in 3 to 1 in 7 will later develop a breast cancer.

Communicating risk

Risks are not additive. The single greatest risk factor is predominant; this is frequently family history.

It is also often important for women to know that the baseline risk of 10–12% is for women who live to be 85 years old, and, actually, the risk of a women aged 30–50 years is only 1 in 1,000/year, which equates to a 2% aggregate risk. Even doubling this with various inherited or acquired risk factors still gives an absolute risk in this age group of only 4%, which is much less than many women realize.

Risk assessment and management for higher risk women are discussed in Chapter 24.

Further reading

Nagtegaal I, Allgood P, Duffy S, *et al.* (2011). Prognosis and pathology of screen-detected carcinomas: how different are they? *Cancer* **117,** 1360–8.

Beral Y; Million Women Study Collaborators (2003). Breast cancer and hormone-replacement therapy in the Million Women Study. *Lancet* **362,** 419–27.

Beral V, Bull D, Reeves G; Million Women Study Collaborators (2005). Endometrial cancer and hormone-replacement therapy in the Million Women study. *Lancet* **365,** 1543–51.

Sweetland S, Beral V, Balkwill A, *et al.* (2012). Venous thromboembolism risk in relation to use of different types of post-menopausal hormone therapy in a large prospective study. *J Thromb Haemost* [Epub ahead of print].

The NHS Breast Screening Programme. Available at: http://www.cancerscreening.nhs.uk/breastscreen/

NICE guidance. Available at: http://www.nice.org.uk/

Familial breast cancer guidance. Available at: http://www.nice.org.uk/CG41

The Association of Breast Surgery. Available at: http://www.associationofbreastsurgery.org.uk/

Chapter 6

Breast assessment: making the diagnosis

Breast clinics

Patients referred to a breast clinic should have their clinical and imaging investigations performed in one visit. This allows the vast majority of symptomatic referrals to be clinically assessed, imaged, reassured, and discharged in one visit. Patients requiring a core biopsy will need a return clinic visit, at which the breast care nurse can, if necessary, be scheduled to be present. Patients having a core biopsy should be advised that their triple assessment results will be discussed in an MDM prior to their next visit. In order to improve the experience for patients, many units have set up clinics for specific issues:

- Young women clinics (<35 years) where there is a low risk of cancer. These clinics will invariably need U/S support.
- Breast pain clinics, focusing on education and coping strategies.
- Family history/high risk clinics centred on risk assessment, genetic counselling, and, occasionally, genetic analysis.
- In addition, most units allow rapid access appointments for women with recurrent problems (e.g. breast cysts and breast abscesses). These appointments are generally accessed through the breast care nurse.

Targets and quality assurance

Patients seen within the NHS need to be managed in accordance with the latest NHS diagnostic and treatment targets and the ABS and NHSBSP symptomatic and screen-detected cancer assessment guidelines and QA standards. So patients need to be seen and treated within certain time frames. It is important that the time frames set can change, as they are often dictated by outside influences rather than clinical need. The underlying feature is to try to reduce the period of anxiety that a patient goes through, having found a worrying sign or symptom in the breast.

Common targets include:

- >93% of symptomatic patients should be seen within 2 weeks of referral date from the GP.
- >96% of patients diagnosed with breast cancer should have treatment within 32 days.
- >85% of patients should have treatment within 2 months (64 days) of referral from the GP.

Primary care referrals

Patients with breast symptoms account for 15% of GP consultations. Breast cancer is the common fear. Breast cancer is not an immediately life-threatening disease, so urgent referral and treatment is unlikely to influence the outcome; nevertheless, prompt diagnosis and treatment can do much to alleviate anxiety.

Over the last 10 years, the focus has been on prioritizing breast referrals into urgent (symptoms/signs suggestive of cancer—to be seen within 2 weeks) and non-urgent (wait up to 13 weeks). However, breast cancer can present with any breast symptom or sign. Prioritization using this system resulted in 30% of cancers being referred through the non-urgent route; in addition, women in the non-urgent group suffered anxiety until they were told their breasts were healthy. Consequently, the referral emphasis has changed to rapid assessment for all breast patients: this alleviates anxiety for all and reduces the wait for diagnosis and treatment if a cancer is detected.

Referral guidelines

These are a useful way of providing GPs and practice nurses with a quick and ready guidance on breast symptoms and when to refer. The guidelines can also be an educational tool for patients, as many patients can be reassured their symptoms and signs are not suggestive of cancer, even if a formal breast assessment is recommended. See Further reading at the end of this chapter for a link to referral guidelines.

The following is an example of a referral guideline for GPs.

Referral criteria for rapid diagnostic symptomatic breast clinic

- <5% of breast cancers occur in women under 40 years.
- <35 years 'whose symptoms/signs are highly suggestive of breast cancer'.

Signs of breast cancer

- **Lump** with dimpling/ulceration.
- **Nipple retraction (new),** distortion, ulceration (unilateral).
- **Others:** change in skin contour, *peau d'orange*, dimpling, and fungation.

Lumps

Please do not needle a lump with no recent/proven history of cysts.

- **Discrete lump:** lumps in post-menopausal women are cancers until proven otherwise.
- **Asymmetrical, discrete, nodularity**: that persists and does not change with cycle.
- **Post-menopausal abscess/infection**: refer for urgent treatment and investigation.

Nipple discharge

Multiduct or multicoloured discharge is innocent duct ectasia.

- Any post-menopausal discharge.

- **Bloodstained** (85% of bloody nipple discharge is benign, e.g. intraduct papilloma).
- **Persistent:** single duct discharge, especially if watery.
- **Excessive**: discharge sufficient to stain clothes (i.e. socially embarrassing).
- **'Eczema':** Paget's ulcerates the nipple, then the areola. Eczema usually affects the areola only.

Pain

Less than 5% of breast cancers **present** with pain and no lump.

- If associated with a lump (usually benign breast changes or cyst).
- Intractable (first, try reassurance, well-supporting bra, dietary and lifestyle changes).
- Unilateral, persistent (>3 months) pain in post-menopausal women.

Women who can be managed by GP/practice nurse

- **Starting HRT**: mammography is not indicated.
- **The majority of women under 30 years:** especially with cyclical, tender, lumpy breasts or **symmetrical** nodularity, with no focal or discrete abnormality.
- **The majority of breast pain**: explain hormonal nature, but exclude musculoskeletal causes.
- **Most nipple discharge:** especially if multiduct/multicoloured.
- **Most family history:** asymptomatic women with average risk.
- **Simple lactational sepsis** that responds to antibiotics.

Common symptoms and signs

The common presenting symptoms seen in the breast clinic are:

- Discrete lumps.
- Lumpiness.
- Pain both cyclical and non-cyclical.
- Nipple discharge.
- Skin/nipple changes.

Patients may present with one, or a combination, of these. Pain accompanied by lumpiness, or what is perceived as a lump, is probably the most frequent presentation in clinic. Although most ladies attending fear they have breast cancer, the reality is that only about one patient in 10–15 attending a standard breast clinic will have breast cancer.

Triple assessment

This consists of:

- Clinical history and examination of the breast.
- Breast imaging.
- Pathological assessment of a biopsy.

Tips for the trainee

Triple assessment is the mainstay of breast assessment, minimizing the chance of missing a breast cancer and allowing treatment planning for those cancers that are identified. Each unit will have its own protocols for breast triple assessment; ask if these are available, and, at your first clinic, ask if you can sit in and watch someone senior do the first few assessments.

Try to follow a patient through the whole process of triple assessment in order to see it from the patient's perspective; see the rest of the unit, and introduce yourself to the whole team.

Triple assessment scores

In order to bring some objectivity to triple assessment, each modality is scored 1 to 5, outlined as follows:

- P—palpability (clinical assessment).
- M—mammography.
- U—U/S.
- B—biopsy.
- C—cytology.

where:

1 = normal appearance.
2 = consistent with a benign lesion.
3 = atypical or indeterminate appearance, probably benign.
4 = suspicious of malignancy.
5 = consistent with malignancy.

NOTE: a score of 1 may also indicate inadequate assessment so needs to be interpreted with caution. For example, this may occur if a needle does not hit its target.

The importance of concordance

Not all cancers present as discrete lumps or with classical clinical or radiological features; this is increasingly so, as women become more breast aware and present with early-stage disease. Similarly, not all cancers are visualized on mammography, so the appropriate use of all three modalities, together with agreement (concordance) between the scores, will reduce, **but not eliminate,** the chance of missing a cancer. The cancer most commonly 'missed' is lobular; clinical and radiological signs can be subtle.

The most common cause of a delay (and subsequent litigation) in breast cancer diagnosis is failure to use triple assessment properly or failure to recognize non-concordance. This is usually due to poor departmental procedures rather than poor individual competence.

No definitive cancer treatment should be undertaken, unless at least two of the three triple assessment modalities are positive for cancer, one of which must be a pathological assessment, usually core biopsy. A false positive diagnosis of breast cancer is rare, but, when it occurs, it can result in devastating consequences for the patient and her family. To avoid this catastrophe, stick to the defined diagnostic pathway.

Clinical assessment

- Introduce yourself; explain your status; make the patient feel at ease.
- Right at the beginning, explain that their case will be discussed with a senior doctor and they may be reviewed by that doctor.
- Sit down at the patient's level; make eye contact.
- Take a history with the patient clothed or appropriately covered.
- Do so in a calm and confident manner.
- If a patient requests a female or a male doctor, try to accommodate this without feeling offended.

The history

This needs to cover the presenting complaint and risk factors for breast cancer (see Chapter 24) or breast sepsis, along with general health issues that may affect treatment of the underlying problem.

- Age.
- Lump: size, shape, when it appeared, how it was noted, any change.
- Nipple discharge: unilateral/bilateral, single duct/multiduct, spontaneous or on stimulation, colour (watery, yellow, green, brown, purulent, bloodstained, blood), pregnancy/breastfeeding.
- Pain: onset, site, severity, relieving and exacerbating factors, cyclical/not.
- Relationship of symptoms to the menstrual cycle: regularity of menses and any oral contraceptive pill (OCP) or HRT taken, intrauterine contraceptive device (IUCD) *in situ*.
- Previous breast cancer, visits to breast clinic, or breast surgery.
- Previous breast imaging: location, dates, and results.
- Risk factors for breast cancer (see Chapter 24): family history, alcohol, weight.
- Hormonal history: menarche, children, breastfeeding, menopause, HRT/hormonal contraception.
- General health and co-morbidities; smoking is important in breast sepsis (see Chapter 7).

The examination

- Always have a chaperone, regardless of your gender.
- The room and your hands must be warm.
- Explain what you are going to do and why (verbal consent).
- Examine in a consistent manner. There are many breast examination techniques. Develop your own after seeing a few.
- Ask the patient to sit on the side of the couch, facing you, and expose their whole torso, displacing hair or jewellery.
- Ask her to point to the area she is concerned about: the patient's use of hand and fingers will give you a clue as to whether it is a focal or generalized problem. It is not uncommon for patients to admit that they are no longer able to identify it.

Note: a lump is different to each patient. Any asymmetrical area should be taken seriously and should be imaged; the overlying tissue may mask a small lump deep within a dense breast, and lobular cancers can often feel diffuse. Younger, more glandular breasts generally feel more 'nodular' than older atrophic breasts, which contain a higher percentage of fat. Almost any type of breast change could indicate an underlying cancer, although the majority of women in the clinic will actually have benign breast change.

- LOOK for asymmetry, visible lumps, and skin dimpling or *peau d'orange*. Inspect the nipple-areola complex (NAC).
- LOOK for skin dimpling or distortion, as the patient slowly raises both hands above the head (to see the whole of the breast) and then lowers the hands and places them on the hips and presses down (to look for muscle fixation when the pectoralis muscle contracts). Look at the nipples for inversion, retraction, or eczematous change. Look at the arms to exclude lymphoedema in advanced or recurrent breast cancer.
- Lay the patient supine at 30° with a pillow under her head and hands tucked under the head.
- Examine the asymptomatic breast first to gain some idea of the normal texture of the breast. Then, examine the symptomatic side. A common technique is to imagine the breast as a clock and work your way around the clock face from 12 to 12, examining the breast from the outer margin towards the nipple as you go. Do not forget the axillary tail and the NAC.
- FEEL with the flat of the fingers.
- Note the site, size, shape, consistency, surface, and fixation of any lumps.
- Check the axillae and infra- and supraclavicular fossae for enlarged lymph nodes (and note their size, texture, etc.).
- If the patient has noted nipple discharge, ask her to demonstrate it. Note whether it is from one or multiple ducts, the colour, any associated nipple changes, and dipstick for the presence of blood. It is sometimes helpful if you are having difficulty feeling a lump to ask the patient to find it, sometimes they have something very small, but, on other occasions, they are surprised to find that they can no longer feel it!

Record-keeping

- Always record examination findings with a drawing, and score your clinical impression P 1–5.
- Mark the site of patient's concern.
- There are standard ways of illustrating your findings.
- Describe the size of the lesion and its position relative to the clock face of the breast and the distance in cm from the NAC.

Initial discussion

Patients may seek reassurance, but this is often not possible until the histology is available and the triple assessment has been discussed in the MDM. Be honest; if you are not sure, say so. Explain to the patient what the next steps will be and how they will hear the results of any further investigations; this means that, before the patient leaves the clinic, they will have been given an appointment for receiving the results.

Breast imaging

The majority of women attending a diagnostic breast clinic will be offered at least one imaging modality, as clinical examination is a poor discriminator of breast pathology, especially in the dense premenopausal breast. Mammography and U/S are the mainstays of imaging, but the use of magnetic resonance imaging (MRI) and other imaging modalities is increasing. Results are scored as outlined previously, using M for mammography and U for U/S scores. Increasingly, both mammography and U/S are used in conjunction, as a proportion of cancers not visible on mammograms will be visible on U/S. If a patient has a clinical lump or asymmetric finding, but a normal mammogram, it is wise to do an U/S as well. It is unlikely that a cancer will be missed with this approach.

Indications for imaging

Guidance on indications for breast imaging has recently changed. Throughout this book, we will be using the Royal College of Radiology Breast Group guidelines (see Further reading).

Check local protocols, which may vary, particularly over age, but consider the following:

- All women >40 years with any symptom, other than pain alone, are offered bilateral mammography to screen both breasts, ideally with targeted U/S (focused on the symptomatic area).
- Women <40 years with the same indications are offered just targeted U/S.

Request forms must state relevant history, side and site of lesion, and clinical impression, with a diagram.

Mammography

This is the gold standard of breast imaging due to its relatively high sensitivity (95% for symptomatic cancers) and specificity compared to clinical examination or U/S. Two views are normally taken, mediolateral oblique (MLO) and cranio-caudal (CC). The total radiation dose is approximately 1mGy (see Fig. 6.1).

Advantages

- 'Screening' of patients attending the breast clinic with a variety of symptoms as outlined (to identify micro-calcifications and small occult cancers).
- Mandatory prior to conservative breast surgery to exclude a second clinically occult cancer in either breast.
- To accurately localize a small or impalpable cancer for excision.

Disadvantages

- Requires breast compression between two plates, which can be uncomfortable.
- Less sensitive in women under age of 40 due to increased background breast density.

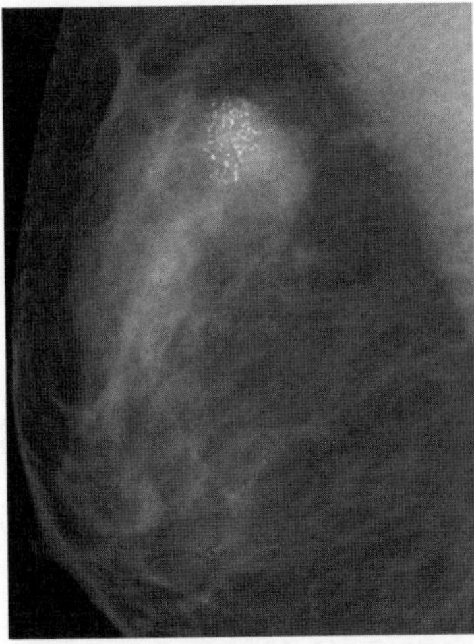

Fig. 6.1 Mediolateral oblique mammogram showing malignant micro-calcification, characteristic of ductal carcinoma *in situ*. Reproduced with permission from 'The Oxford Textbook of Medicine' 5th edn., edited by David A. Warrell, Timothy M. Cox, John D. Firth, copyright 2010 Oxford University Press.

Ultrasound (U/S)

High-frequency sound waves are directed through the breast, and reflections from different tissue components are detected and turned into images (see Fig. 6.2). The specificity of distinguishing a cyst from a solid lesion is almost 100%, and an experienced operator can be both sensitive and specific.

Advantages

- Useful for all palpable lumps and usually the sole imaging technique for women less than 40 years.
- Forms part of the preoperative assessment of the axilla in ladies with breast cancer (any abnormal nodes have FNA or core under U/S guidance).
- No radiation.
- Not uncomfortable.
- Allows accurate sizing of lesions (at first visit and after neoadjuvant chemotherapy or hormonal therapy; see Chapter 13).
- Can distinguish discrete lumps from areas of nodularity in young women.
- The majority of core biopsies are performed under U/S guidance.

If a breast cancer is detected, simultaneously U/S the axilla and use U/S to guide FNAC of any enlarged axillary lymph nodes. This may allow most appropriate use of axillary clearance and sentinel lymph node techniques.

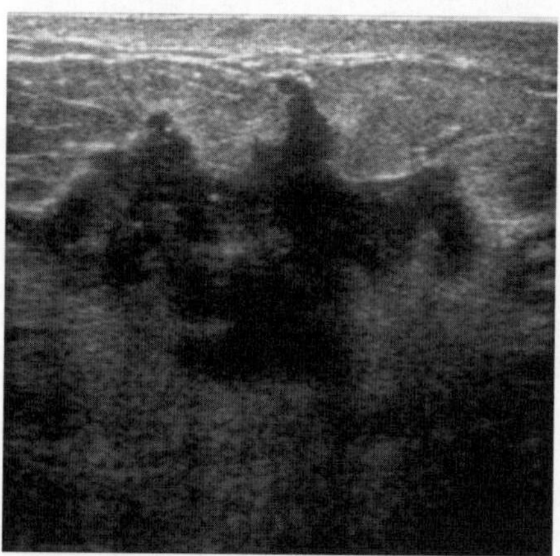

Fig. 6.2 Ultrasound scan showing the characteristic appearance of an invasive cancer with micro-calcification. Reproduced with permission from 'The Oxford Textbook of Medicine' 5th edn., edited by David A. Warrell, Timothy M. Cox, John D. Firth, copyright 2010 Oxford University Press.

Disadvantages

- Operator-dependent.
- Not useful to visualize micro-calcifications.
- Poor 'screening tool', less sensitive than mammography.
- Less easy for subsequent radiologists to comment on images, as it is a 'live image' and user-dependent.

MRI

Based on the nuclear spin of molecules when subjected to a strong magnetic field. Useful to image the augmented breast, to assess multifocality (particularly in lobular cancers), or in screening of young women with a strong family history of breast cancer. However, specificity is low; cost is high, and availability may be limited, so **check local protocols.**

Pathology

Wide bore needle (core) biopsy

Pathology

- In general, random needling of a generally lumpy area should be avoided. Histopathology should be reserved for a discrete solid lesion on clinical examination and/or imaging, as, with imaging, there will often be local protocols.
- Pathology request forms must state relevant history, side and site of lesion, and clinical impression, usually with a diagram.
- Results are scored C1–5 for cytology and B1–B5a/b for histopathology. B5a denotes *in situ* carcinoma; B5b denotes an invasive carcinoma, and B5c a carcinoma with microinvasion.
- Because histopathology can report on the architecture of the lesion as well as cellular appearance, core biopsy has now replaced FNAC. Simple cysts, which have a typical appearance on U/S, do not need to be aspirated, unless they are uncomfortable. If they are aspirated, clear fluid does not need to be sent to pathology. However, bloody aspirates can be sent to exclude a necrotic cancer with cystic degeneration or an intracystic carcinoma or papilloma. Similarly, any residual lump left after cyst aspiration should be subjected to histological analysis.

Fine-needle aspiration cytology (FNAC)

Advantages

- Quick and easy to perform.
- Results available in about 30 minutes (for one-stop clinic).
- Samples a large area.

Disadvantages

- Information is limited to benign or malignant. Cannot distinguish DCIS from invasive cancer.
- Results are dependent upon the operator doing the FNAC and the cytologist interpreting it.
- Not useful in assessing micro-calcification.

Wide-bore needle (core) biopsy

Advantages

- Gives information on morphology, grade, hormone receptor status, Her-2 status which helps in treatment planning.
- Biopsies are larger than FNAC, so more of the lesion is sampled.

Disadvantages

- More bruising.
- Results take longer (24 to 48 hours).

Punch biopsy

Used to biopsy skin lesions, e.g. to differentiate eczema from Paget's disease of the nipple and to diagnose or exclude malignancy in skin nodules. Once again, this takes 24 to 48 hours for the histology result.

Nipple discharge dipstick and cytology

Fluid expressed from the nipple can be dipsticked for the presence of blood and can be smeared onto a slide and sent for cytology. Rarely useful to identify pathological discharge containing blood cells or malignant cells.

Open/surgical biopsy

Rarely needed to make a diagnosis since over 95% of cancers are confirmed preoperatively using triple assessment. Only used when repeat biopsy is not possible or unlikely to be helpful (usually for small screen-detected lesions). Generally involves wire-guided techniques. Microdochectomy and central duct excision procedures for bloody or troublesome nipple discharge also fall into this category.

Miscellaneous investigations

These depend upon the mode of presentation of the patient.

- Blood tests
  - May be useful in the investigation of gynaecomastia (see Chapter 9).
- Microbiology
  - Try to get a culture from any breast sepsis prior to commencing antibiotics.
- Staging investigations
  - Locally advanced breast cancers or patients with symptoms that raise the question of metastatic disease may require bone scan and CT chest, abdomen, and pelvis.

At the end of the consultation, it should be possible either to reassure the patient that their problem is benign or to warn them of the possibility of a cancer.

If tissue has been taken for pathology, all the results—clinical, radiological, and imaging—should be discussed at the diagnostic MDT at which a plan of management can be formulated. Avoid making spur-of-the minute decisions at the end of clinic, as this often leads to disaster and mistakes being made.

Further reading

National GP guidelines and breast screening guidelines. Available at: http://www.cancerscreening.nhs.uk/breastscreen/publications

Willett AM, Michell JM, Lee MJR (2010). Best practice diagnostic guidelines for patients presenting with breast symptoms. Available at: http://www.associationofbreastsurgery.org.uk/publications-guidelines/guidelines.aspx

The Royal College of Radiology Breast Group guidelines. Available at: http://www.rcrbreastgroup.com/Documents/BBCDiagnosticGuidelines.pdf

Surgical guidelines for the management of breast cancer. Association of Breast Surgery at BASO, 2009. *EJSO* S1–22. Available at: http://www.ejso.com

NICE guidance management of early and locally advanced breast cancer (2009). Available at: http://www.nice.org.uk/nicemedia/pdf/CG80NICEGuideline.pdf

Chapter 7

Benign breast problems and their management

Overview

Benign breast disease forms the bulk of outpatient diagnostic referrals in breast clinics. It encompasses a diverse range of problems, ranging from congenital abnormalities, physiological aberrations, and infections. Few, if any, are associated with any serious risk of disease; nevertheless, they cause immense anxiety because, in the perception of many women, any breast symptom is synonymous with cancer. Their management requires explanation and reassurance to dispel patients' fears.

Guidance on indications for breast imaging has recently changed. Throughout this book, we will be using the Royal College of Radiology Breast Group guidelines (see Further reading).

Congenital problems

These encompass a variety of problems that result in an abnormal appearance in the external appearance of the breast.

Athelia

This is the complete absence of the nipple and is usually unilateral.

Polythelia

This refers to accessory or supernumerary nipples which occur along the milk (mid-clavicular) line. Incidence is 1–2%. These are associated with accessory breast tissue and renal anomalies. Supernumerary breasts are defined as accessory structures that produce milk. Most occur in the axillo-pectoral region and are generally noticed in the second to third pregnancy. Local excision is usually curative but should not be performed whilst women are still lactating due to risk of fistula formation. Malignancy has occasionally been reported in accessory nipples.

Amastia

This is a congenital absence of breast tissue, but the nipple is still present. Hypoplasia of one or both breasts is a more common finding and is associated with mitral valve prolapse.

Poland's syndrome

Occurring at an incidence of approximately 1:7,000 to 1:100,000, this syndrome describes an absence/underdevelopment of the pectoralis muscle, cutaneous ipsilateral syndactyly, and hypoplasia of the breast. All three features need not be present for a diagnosis of Poland's syndrome. The cause is unknown but may result from an interruption to the embryonic blood supply of the subclavian region.

Other associated signs: brachydactyly, renal anomalies, liver/biliary tract anomalies, dextrocardia, radial/ulnar agenesis, and upper limb asymmetry.

Management of congenital disorders

Accessory nipples can usually be excised without major cosmetic insult. Other congenital abnormalities present a much greater aesthetic challenge. A wide variety of surgical techniques may need to be employed as staged procedures. They are best managed by a reconstructive team.

Breast development and involution

Breast development and involution occurs throughout life.

- Breast development: occurs in both sexes from about the age of 10. Initially, this development may be asymmetrical. Beware of any surgery on a developing breast, as this can significantly damage the breast bud with consequent long-term deformity.
- Menstruation: the breast undergoes regular changes associated with the menstrual cycle.
- Pregnancy and lactation: causes lobuloalveolar growth and milk production.
- Involution: this process begins from age 30 in nulliparous women. Fat replaces breast tissue, and lobular stroma is replaced by fibrous tissue.

Aberrations of normal development and involution (ANDI)

This describes a group of conditions that are so common they should be considered as normal variations of these physiological processes; however, their symptoms and signs frequently cause anxiety and result in referral for reassurance, if nothing else. They are seen throughout life, starting with menarche, going through early adult life and menstruation to older age and menopause. The classification describes the various changes seen in the breast at those times which result in perceived symptoms and signs.

- Breast development: juvenile hypertrophy, accessory breast tissue, and fibroadenoma.
- Menstruation: fibroadenoma, cyclical nodularity, localized benign nodularity.
- Involution: breast cyst, fibrocystic change, sclerosing lesions (radial scar and complex sclerosing lesions), duct ectasia.

Diagnosis

- Up to 70% of patients referred to a breast clinic will complain of a lump or lumpiness.
- Fig. 7.1 demonstrates the frequency of common breast lumps with increasing age.
- Clinical assessment, followed by radiological and pathological assessment as required, will result in the diagnosis of these common breast lumps.

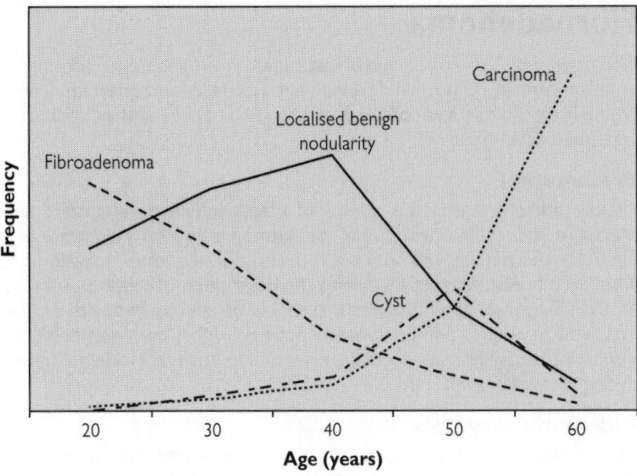

Fig. 7.1 The frequency and age at presentation of the most common breast lumps.

Fibroadenoma

Fibroadenomas are not benign breast tumours but should be considered as an abnormality of normal development. Fibroadenomas develop from a whole breast lobule and contain a combination of proliferating epithelium and connective tissue.

Presentation

Usually present during the period of breast lobule development and, therefore, are commonest during the late teens and early twenties (see Fig. 7.1). The patient will notice a rubbery, discrete, often mobile lump within the breast which gives rise to the description of these as a 'breast mouse'. Diagnosis of a fibroadenoma should be approached with caution in a woman who is peri- or post-menopausal. Most common presentation is with a painless symptomatic breast lump or as an incidental finding during breast imaging.

Differential diagnosis

Fibroadenomas contain stroma of low cellularity and regular cytology. Phyllodes tumours are a mesenchymal variant and have a spectrum of stromal cellularity and varying degrees of atypia.

Natural history

Patients under 40 can be advised that the majority of fibroadenomas remain static in size; approximately 10% will enlarge, and one-third will get smaller or resolve over a 2-year period. Although malignancy can very rarely develop within a fibroadenoma, they should not be seen as having any malignant tendency, and this should be stressed to the patient. Pregnancy can occasionally result in rapid growth.

Assessment

Clinical assessment of a fibroadenoma will reveal a well-defined and firm, but not hard, lesion that is mobile within the breast. All lumps require clinical assessment and imaging. Imaging: if woman <40 years, use ultrasound alone, if >40 years mammography and ultrasound. Ultrasound-guided core biopsy should be performed on all lumps, unless the following criteria are all met:

- Patient under 25 years of age.
- Ultrasound reveals benign features of a fibroadenoma (smooth, well-defined outline, ellipsoid shape, fewer than four gentle lobulations).
- No significant family history of breast cancer.

Management

Simple reassurance is sufficient for the vast majority of patients. Surgical excision in the form of enucleation can be performed for large (>4cm) or enlarging fibroadenomas, or if there is any histological concern from the triple assessment. Surgical excision should be performed, using either a peri-areolar or an inframammary subglandular approach to minimize visible scarring. Vacuum-assisted excision under ultrasound control is now becoming the method of choice for smaller lesions when the patient requests removal.

Giant fibroadenomas

Defined as fibroadenomas over 5cm in diameter or 500g in weight. Giant fibroadenomas have a bimodal presentation, peaking in adolescence and peri-menopausally. More frequent in Asian and African populations. Treatment is with local excision/enucleation, using an inframammary approach. These can sometimes be drug-induced by anti-epileptic drugs, such as phenytoin and ciclosporin.

Phyllodes tumour

Phyllodes tumours are less common than fibroadenomas (ratio 1:50), and their aetiology is unknown. These tumours represent a spectrum from benign lesions (common) through to malignant sarcomas which rarely metastasize. In contrast to fibroadenomas, phyllodes tumours should be excised with a surrounding margin of normal breast tissue in a similar fashion to a carcinoma. Approximately 20% of these lesions will recur locally within the breast, requiring further wide local excision. It is important to discuss these lesions preoperatively in the MDM.

Breast cysts

Breast cysts affect approximately 7% of peri-menopausal women and can rarely be found in men. Breast involution occurs in the peri-menopausal period, as female hormone levels begin to fall, coinciding with the production of breast cysts. Breast cysts account for 15% of all breast lumps and affect women aged 40–60 (see Fig. 7.1). Women taking hormone replacement therapy (HRT) may develop breast cysts well after their natural menopause.

Presentation

Cysts may be found symptomatically by the patient as a hard lump or incidentally through the screening programme. Patients commonly have multiple cysts affecting both breasts. Examination will reveal a mobile lump, extremely well-defined and smooth, at times slightly compressible in nature. They often enlarge very rapidly during the menstrual cycle, causing great alarm. It is common for patients to say that they appeared overnight.

Differential diagnosis

- Galactocele (encapsulated collection of milk within the obstructed duct of a lactating breast).
- Liquefied haematoma.
- Carcinoma.
- Oil cyst secondary to fat necrosis.

Management

All suspected cysts should have clinical and imaging assessment, no matter how many times the patient has previously presented with breast cysts.

Imaging

Women over 40 should have mammography and ultrasound performed. Women under age 40 should have ultrasound alone. Ultrasound should demonstrate a thin-walled, well-defined fluid-filled lesion. Ultrasound features suggestive of a risk of malignancy include a thickened wall, thick internal septations, mixed solid and fluid composition, and an imaging classification of indeterminate.

Pathological assessment

- Complex/radiologically indeterminate cysts should be core-biopsied and results discussed in a multidisciplinary breast team meeting.
- Simple symptomatic cysts should be aspirated to dryness under ultrasound control. Green/brown/black serous fluid can be discarded. Bloodstained discharge is a risk factor for an intracystic cancer and requires cytology.
- Asymptomatic cysts with no suspicious clinical or radiological features do not require aspiration or pathological assessment; this includes the majority of screen-detected cysts.

Treatment

Women with simple cysts can be reassured but should be forewarned about the risk of developing further cysts in the future. Simple cysts that recur can be repeatedly aspirated and do not have an increased risk of cancer, provided there are no suspicious features on imaging. Breast cysts are not a risk factor for cancer; however, as both breast cancers and breast cysts are common in this age group, each new subsequent lump should be assessed in a one-stop breast clinic. Women taking HRT should be advised that stopping treatment might prevent subsequent cyst development.

Complex cysts should have core biopsy performed. If this is non-diagnostic, a surgical diagnostic excision biopsy should be undertaken.

Other common benign breast lumps

Hamartoma

This is a disorganized overgrowth of normal breast tissue; one element of the breast tissue will usually predominate. These are benign lumps but can grow progressively. Hamartomas do not have distinctive histopathological features, hence diagnosis requires correlation between clinical, radiological, and pathological findings (see Further reading).

Presentation

Symptomatic, soft to firm, well-defined mass. The initial clinical diagnosis is usually of a fibroadenoma.

Management

Ultrasound (plus mammography if >40 years of age), along with clinical correlation, can safely diagnose the majority of hamartomas. Clinically (P2) and radiologically benign (U2 and M1/2) lesions do not require biopsy. If any doubt exists about the nature of the lesion or if there is any clinical/radiological discrepancy, an ultrasound-guided core biopsy should be performed. Hamartomas cannot be diagnosed from a pathological specimen; multidisciplinary team correlation is essential.

Surgery

Excision of these benign lesions should be offered for symptomatic patients. Excision should be performed with a cosmetic inframammary or peri-areolar incision. A narrow margin should be taken, although local recurrence is rare.

Fat necrosis

Fat necrosis is a partial necrosis of adipose tissue with an associated inflammatory response.

Causes

Trauma (from minor knocks to the breast to a seat belt-induced injury), surgery, radiotherapy, mammography, iatrogenic injections to breast (e.g. patent blue).

Presentation

Initially presents with a firm, tender lump within the breast, often mimicking a carcinoma and often with a history of trauma and extensive bruising. May be associated with an inflammatory response, causing a red, hot, oedematous breast, sometimes associated with nipple retraction. Subsequent scarring within the breast may cause parenchymal distortion. Over time, the acute inflammatory response will settle, and fat begins to liquefy and the lump softens and resolves. Superficial fat necrosis following surgery may present with fatty discharge from the wound.

Imaging

Fat necrosis can also simulate a carcinoma radiologically. Ultrasound (and mammography if >40 years of age), together with a clinical picture, will diagnose the majority of fat necrosis lesions. If any doubt exists about the nature of the lesion or if there is any clinical/radiological discrepancy, an ultrasound-guided core biopsy should be performed. The core biopsy appearance can also be equivocal (B3/B4), requiring repeat core or occasionally open biopsy.

Treatment

It is vital to exclude carcinoma. Having done that, no specific treatment is required other than reassurance of the benign nature of the lesion. Lesions resolve with time but may leave residual fibrous scarring.

Mondor's syndrome

Mondor's syndrome is a superficial thrombophlebitic process in the subcutaneous veins of the thoraco-abdominal wall.

Presentation

The syndrome presents as a superficial, cord-like thrombophlebitis. Commonly affects the superior epigastric, thoracoepigastric, and lateral thoracic veins as far inferiorly as the umbilicus. Associated findings are pain, erythema, pruritus, and rarely fever. Occasionally associated with breast malignancy. Mammography should be performed for women over 40.

Causation

Primarily induced by trauma, including breast surgery, physical activity, breast infection, pendulous breasts, and rarely breast cancer.

Natural history

The palpable thrombophlebitis is a self-limiting condition, resolving in 2 weeks to 6 months. The pain of the acute inflammatory reaction subsides within 10 days.

Management

Reassurance, rest, breast support, and analgesia form the mainstay of treatment. Oral or topical non-steroidal anti-inflammatories are helpful in the acute inflammatory phase.

Duct ectasia and periductal mastitis

Duct ectasia is part of normal breast ageing and is common towards the menopause. Periductal mastitis is the inflammatory condition which may complicate this and may go on to form a subareolar abscess. However, periductal mastitis can be seen in younger women before ectasia has developed and, in these circumstances, is frequently associated with smoking.

Clinical features

- Nipple discharge: clear/coloured, thick/thin, occasionally bloodstained.
- Breast abscesses: commonly peri-areolar.
- Inflammatory breast mass: often chronic.
- Nipple retraction.
- Mammary duct fistula: associated with recurrent abscesses and nipple inversion.
- Mastalgia.
- Eczema: associated with chronic nipple discharge.

Pathology

Duct ectasia is characterized by dilated ducts, extending 2–3cm behind the nipple. Periductal inflammation causes shortening and retraction of the ducts; this may be associated with abscess formation.

Microbiology

Some masses demonstrate no bacterial growth. Common organisms found are a mixture of aerobes and anaerobes (*Staphylococcus epidermidis* and *aureus*, Peptostreptococci, Bacteroides, Proteus).

Causation

Clinical syndrome may be related, in some women, to obstructed ducts or pre-existing nipple inversion. Smokers are more likely to have severe disease with fistula formation, anaerobic growth, and abscess formation.

Assessment

All breast masses require triple assessment to establish diagnosis. Ultrasound will demonstrate dilated ducts associated with duct ectasia. Microbiological assessment of any fluid aspirated may guide treatment.

Management

- Non-painful mass: observe initially, as it may resolve.
- Painful mass: microbiological assessment. Treat with broad-spectrum antibiotics, e.g. co-amoxiclav, NOT flucloxacillin.
- Abscess: repeated ultrasound-guided aspirations and broad-spectrum antibiotics. Open drainage if fistulating through skin.

Surgery

- Excision biopsy: for retro-areolar mass not responding to antibiotics.
- Correction of nipple inversion: can result in a worsening of cosmesis. Patient must be aware of risk of nipple necrosis, loss of sensation, inability to breastfeed, and recurrence of the inversion.

- Fistula surgery: fistulectomy can be performed in a young patient with a single tract. Older patients and those with complex disease or purulent discharge require total duct excision. The wound can be closed by primary or secondary intention.

Recurrent infection following surgery can be caused by: persistent abscess cavity, persistent proximal or distal ducts, nipple inversion, early pregnancy, factitial disease, or contralateral disease. Recurrent problems are common in smokers.

Breast infections: mastitis and abscesses

Mastitis is defined as an infection of the breast parenchyma whereas an abscess is a localized collection of pus within the parenchyma, usually surrounded by an area of mastitis.

Aetiology

Breast abscesses commonly occur in two distinct age groups (see Table 7.1).

- Lactational: affects 3% lactating women, 80% in the first month post-partum. Almost exclusively skin-derived infection arising from cracking of the nipple. Can be reduced with good nipple hygiene and skin care.
- Non-lactational: secondary to periductal mastitis/duct ectasia, age 35–55, more common in smokers. Commonest site is subareolar.

Breast infections can be caused by atypical infections, especially in an immunocompromised patient; these include *Mycobacterium tuberculosis*, fungi, filariasis, hydatid, Pseudomonas, or mumps.

Presentation

Examination reveals a red, hot, swollen, indurated, and tender breast. Due to the density and engorgement of a lactational breast, it can be difficult to clinically determine the presence of an abscess within an area of mastitis. Ultrasound demonstrates the presence of any underlying abscess cavity.

Management

- Antibiotics.
- Drainage: ultrasound-guided aspiration of an abscess cavity should be performed under local anaesthetic. Serial ultrasound-guided aspirations will be required over several weeks. Surgical drainage is only used for abscesses that have breached overlying necrotic skin (see Further reading). Surgical drainage should be avoided because it may leave unsightly scars and increase the risk of subsequent fistula formation. This latter complication is more common with abscesses related to periductal mastitis than lactation.
- Lactational abscess: women must be reassured to continue to breastfeed or to express milk to avoid an engorged breast full of milk which makes an excellent culture broth. The *S. aureus* contaminated milk will not harm their baby.
- Non-lactational abscess: these infections are persistent and can be difficult to clear, especially if the patient continues to smoke. Offer Stop Smoking support.

Table 7.1 A demonstration of the two common types of breast abscess: lactational and non-lactational

	Lactational	**Non-lactational**
Common organisms	*S. aureus*, *S. epidermidis*	Mixed aerobic/ anaerobic (Bacteroides, *S. aureus*, *S. epidermidis*, Peptostreptococcus)
First-line antibiotic	Flucloxacillin	Co-amoxiclav
Penicillin allergy	Erythromycin	Erythromycin

The aetiology and flora of the infections must be appreciated to instigate the appropriate antibiotic therapy.

Granulomatous mastitis

Granulomatous mastitis is a rare, benign, inflammatory condition of the breast, often without an obvious cause.

Aetiology

Multiple aetiologies have been suggested, including tuberculosis (TB), sarcoidosis, foreign body reaction, and parasitic infections. In the majority of cases, no cause is found.

Epidemiology

Most common in third and fourth decades of life and is associated with recent pregnancy and lactation. Uncommon in nulliparous women.

Presentation

A breast mass is the most common clinical finding. The mass may penetrate the skin to form an ulcer or fistula, pucker the skin, or be tethered to underlying muscle. Parenchymal and nipple distortion, and axillary lymphadenopathy may be present; these findings may suggest a breast carcinoma.

A full history of infectious diseases/contacts should be taken, including TB contacts. Associated with autoimmune disease, including Wegener's granulomatosis, erythema nodosum, and polyarteritis nodosa.

Most patients with breast infections will be smokers. The presence of an apparently infectious lesion in a non-smoker should alert the clinician to the possibility that this might be granulomatous mastitis.

Imaging

Mammographic findings include focal asymmetric density and parenchymal distortion. Ultrasound examination may reveal focal, homogeneous enhancing masses and abscess formation.

Diagnosis

Differentiating granulomatous mastitis from carcinoma can be difficult and may require ultrasound-guided biopsy of the lesion. Further pathological assessment may be required using vacuum-assisted or, rarely, open biopsy.

Further investigation

Microbiological assessment is essential of any abscess fluid and of biopsies taken of the mass. Prolonged TB culture and PCR analysis may be helpful. Corynebacterium may be isolated.

Treatment

Granulomatous mastitis probably represents a spectrum of diseases, causing a similar clinical and pathological picture. Multiple treatments may be required for clinical cure. Optimal treatment is controversial. Discussion at the MDM is important, and getting a second MDM opinion may be helpful. Many patients with an obviously 'infected' breast will become concerned if 'nothing' appears to be done.

Note that patients need careful explanation of the benefits of observation. In the majority of patients, masterly inactivity and open access to the clinic when they are concerned is often the best option; however, if active treatment is undertaken, the following options exist.

- Anti-microbials: in the presence of a proven infection, prolonged anti-microbial treatment (2–6 weeks) is required.
- Wide excision: wide local excision, with margins clear of inflammatory tissue, may give long-term cure but often at the expense of cosmesis. This is a very controversial approach; some would advise avoiding surgery at all costs.
- Steroid treatment: prednisolone 10–30mg/day for up to 8 weeks has been used prior to surgery and after excision. Prolonged use of steroids may help prevent multiple deforming operations.
- Immunosuppression: weekly low-dose oral methotrexate has shown benefit in a small number of cases resistant to steroid therapy.

Complications

Major complications include recurrence and fistula formation which is often the result of premature surgery. Recurrence rates are up to 50% following surgical excision/steroid therapy. Excision of the recurrence and further steroid treatment may be needed. The mastitis is characterized by long-term resolution, often over several years.

Radial scar and complex sclerosing lesions

Definition

Radial scar and complex sclerosing lesions represent areas of benign myoepithelial proliferation with or without micro-calcification. Histologically, they are characterized by a fibroelastic core with entrapped ducts and surrounded by radiating ducts and lobules. Sclerosing lesions <1cm in diameter are termed radial scars and those >1cm complex sclerosing lesions.

Presentation

Sclerosing lesions are asymptomatic and are detected on mammography, most commonly as part of the National Health Service Breast Screening Programme. The detection of these lesions has increased dramatically since the introduction of population-based mammographic screening, with an incidence of one in every 500 women screened. Clinical examination may occasionally reveal a mass lesion.

Imaging

Sclerosing lesions require careful assessment because, radiologically, they can mimic carcinoma. Common features on mammography include:

- The presence of a central radiolucency.
- Radiating long spicules.
- Radiolucent linear structures parallel to spicules.
- Absence of a mass lesion or skin changes.
- Varying appearance in different projections.

Pathological assessment

All sclerosing lesions require careful pathological assessment to exclude a malignancy. This can be achieved using multiple core biopsies or vacuum-assisted sampling mammotome. If diagnostic doubt remains following radiologically guided biopsy, an open diagnostic biopsy should be performed.

Management

Sclerosing lesions alone are entirely benign and do not increase future breast cancer risk. Sclerosing lesions can harbour atypical hyperplasia and ductal carcinoma *in situ*. Due to the risk of an associated atypical lesion, sclerosing lesions should either undergo a diagnostic excision biopsy or, following benign biopsies, should undergo mammographic surveillance.

Breast pain (mastalgia)

Breast pain is the commonest presenting symptom in the breast clinic, affecting up to 50% of patients. Patients present with pain alone or a painful lumpiness.

History

Association with the menstrual cycle differentiates breast pain into cyclical and non-cyclical. True breast pain must be differentiated from pain referred from the chest wall or other organs. Typically, true breast pain increases in the days prior to menstruation and subsides once menstruation has started. Daily breast pain charts are useful for confirming to both the patient and the health professional the nature and timing of the symptoms. A thorough history of the nature of pain, causative or related factors, hormonal medication, and other musculoskeletal conditions will help to exclude non-breast conditions.

Examination

Routine breast and axillary examination should be performed. The chest wall adjacent to the lateral fold of the breast should also be carefully examined with the patient lying on their side. Focal musculoskeletal tenderness in this region commonly causes referred breast pain. Examination of chest wall, abdomen, shoulders, and spine may identify other potential causes of non-cyclical breast pain requiring further evaluation.

Causation

Cyclical mastalgia

- Commonest type of mastalgia.
- Can be focal or global breast pain, unilateral or bilateral.

Non-cyclical mastalgia

- Chest wall causes: localized musculoskeletal tenderness, Tietze's syndrome (costochondritis).
- Focal point tenderness within breast.
- Diffuse breast tenderness.
- Non-breast causes: spondylosis, gallstones, lung disease, exogenous oestrogens, thoracic outlet syndrome.

Imaging

Imaging is only required where there is associated or incidental, focal clinical signs in the breast (localized tenderness, nodularity, swelling, or a lump). The majority of patients will not require any form of imaging.

Management

Information

All patients should receive verbal information and reassurance about the nature of the pain. Patients should be given a written information leaflet. This forms the mainstay of treatment. The risks and benefits of the few therapeutic options should be explained.

Chest wall pain

Musculoskeletal tenderness requires rest and reassurance. Topical or oral anti-inflammatories may provide some relief.

Localized chest wall tenderness

Oral anti-inflammatories. Depot injection of methylprednisolone 40mg and local anaesthetic, repeated as necessary at 6 weeks, provides long-lasting analgesia in 60% of patients.

True breast pain

- Supportive soft, non-underwired bra, particularly useful for pain at night. Bra fitting should be offered within the breast clinic.
- Topical anti-inflammatory application, e.g. ibuprofen gel.
- Endocrine treatments (rarely used): danazol 200mg once per day given in the luteal phase (day 15–25 of cycle) has a response rate of 70% in cyclical and 30% in non-cyclical mastalgia. Significant side effects include weight gain, acne, and hirsutism. Tamoxifen 10mg given in the luteal phase gives long-term pain relief in up to 70% of women. Tamoxifen is, however, unlicensed for breast pain.
- Antidepressants: selective serotonin reuptake inhibitors have limited benefit in some patients.

Nipple discharge

History

Establish the duration, frequency, volume, and colour of nipple discharge. Does it occur spontaneously or only on squeezing; whether bilateral; and whether there are any other associated breast symptoms, particularly a lump or inflammation.

Clinical features

Breast examination should detail nipple inversion and eczematous changes. Asking the patient to express the discharge will determine if it is single or multiple ducts, colour, and the presence of blood. Urinalysis sticks are a useful guide to the presence of blood. Cytology of the discharge is of limited clinical value. Twenty percent of men with nipple discharge have breast cancer.

Features of nipple discharge associated with malignancy

Associated recent nipple inversion, unilateral nipple eczema or nipple change, bloodstained discharge (especially from solitary duct).

Investigation

Bilateral mammography in those over 40. Ultrasound if single-duct discharge or if any palpable abnormality. Punch biopsy for unexplained nipple eczema or ulceration. Serum prolactin in patients with persistent milky discharge.

Causes of nipple discharge

- Multiduct clear galactorrhoea: mechanical stimulation, post-lactational, stress, menopause, menarche, drugs (dopamine blockers, methyldopa, oral contraceptives, metoclopramide), pituitary tumours, bronchogenic carcinoma, hypothyroidism, renal failure.
- Single-duct clear discharge: papilloma.
- Multicoloured discharge: duct ectasia, cysts.
- Bloodstained discharge: duct ectasia, DCIS, invasive carcinoma, pregnancy, papilloma.

Smokers are more likely to have severe disease with fistula formation, anaerobic growth, and abscess formation.

Treatment

- Reassurance and advice to not express the discharge is the mainstay of treatment for women with benign multiduct discharge.
- Microdochectomy: for persistent single-duct discharge, whether clear or bloody. Also perform if papilloma present on ultrasound.
- Total duct excision: bloodstained discharge in woman over 45. Patient choice due to persistent multiduct discharge. Nipple eczema secondary to persistent discharge.

Solitary papilloma

Peak incidence at age 45. Occurs within 5cm of nipple and are generally 2–3mm in diameter. Fifty percent present with bloody/clear discharge; 50% have a palpable lump; 8% contain neoplasia.

Multiple duct papillomas

Less likely to cause discharge. Present with bilateral peripheral lumps. Increased risk of breast carcinoma. Increased risk can be managed with surveillance (little evidence of best way to perform this) or risk-reducing surgery.

Further reading

Tse G, Law BK, Ma TK, *et al.* (2002). Hamartoma of the breast: a clinicopathological review. *J Clin Pathol* **55**, 951–4.

Ocal K, Dag A, Turkmenoglu O, Kara T, Seyit H, Konica K (2010). Granulomatous mastitis: clinical, pathological features and management. *Breast J* **16**,176–82.

Kim J, Tymms KE, Buckingham JM (2003). Methotrexate in the management of granulomatous mastitis. *ANZ J Surg* **73**, 247–9.

Mansel R, Webster D, Sweetland H (2009). *Hughes, Mansel & Webster's Benign disorders and diseases of the breast*, 3e. Saunders Ltd, Philadelphia.

Dixon J (1992). Outpatient treatment of non-lactational breast abscesses. *Br J Surg* **79**, 56–7

Wallis MG, Devakumar R, Hosie KB, James KA, Bishop HM (1993). Complex sclerosing lesions (radial scars) of the breast can be palpable. *Clin Radiol* **48**, 319–20.

Breast Pain Chart at Breast Cancer Care. Available at: http://www.breastcancercare.org.uk/upload/pdf/breast_pain_chart.pdf

The Royal College of Radiology Breast Group guidelines. Available at: http://www.rcrbreastgroup.com/Documents/BBCDiagnosticGuidelines.pdf

Chapter 8

Surgical management of benign breast disease

Breast abscess

See also Chapter 7.

- Requires adequate drainage.
- Delay can lead to breast tissue and skin loss, poor cosmetic result and impede breastfeeding.
- Normally managed by aspiration (ideally under U/S guidance) in the A&E or outpatient setting. Only a small number require formal incision and drainage.
- After aspiration/drainage, consider admission and intravenous antibiotics in systemically unwell women, particularly those on chemotherapy or other immunosuppressive drugs, or those with extensive cellulitis.
- Following complete aspiration or drainage, the patient can be discharged but should return to the breast clinic within 48 hours for review, as many need repeat aspiration and/or further evaluation in non-lactational abscesses to exclude an underlying breast cancer. There is a danger at weekends and public holidays that there will be inappropriately long intervals between aspirations, so suitable arrangement must be made.

If the skin is intact, and the patient consents

- Treat with simple aspiration.
- Apply EMLA® cream to the skin. Going through non-indurated skin is less painful.
- Using a 19G needle, aspirate the abscess, ideally under U/S guidance if an U/S machine, or a friendly radiologist, is available.
- The needle should be inserted parallel to the chest wall to avoid the small chance of a pneumothorax.
- An appropriate volume of 1% lidocaine, or similar local anaesthetic, can be infiltrated into the abscess and the abscess aspirated, with a 'washing' in and out of the local anaesthetic.
- Send a sample of the pus to microbiology.
- Commence appropriate antibiotics, as outlined in Chapter 7.
- Do not insert a needle blindly into a breast with an implant. If you think there is an abscess here, it is possible that the implant will need to be removed to eradicate the infection. Discuss U/S-guided aspiration with a breast radiologist.

If the overlying skin is necrotic or aspiration fails

- Formal incision and drainage under general anaesthesia.
- Remember that drainage will be gravitational when the patient sits or stands. Occasionally, this requires drainage through the inframammary crease.
- Clean the skin with povidone-iodine or chlorhexidine.
- Necrotic skin should be removed with a blade or scissors and a good pair of forceps.
- Locules should be broken down gently, and the cavity should be washed out with saline.

- Send a sample of pus to microbiology and the wall to histopathology.
- The wound can be left open (not sutured) to improve drainage.
- Packing can be minimal (a small wick of Kaltostat®) to reduce discomfort.
- Commence appropriate antibiotics if any residual cellulitis.

Operations on the nipple/major ducts

Microdochectomy

This is the removal of a single duct from the breast, usually performed for single-duct discharge.

Planning

Mark patient standing up (side, intended scar, and possibly duct involved).

Positioning

Supine with arm by side or abducted to 90°.

Scar/incision

Peri-areolar. Avoid going more than halfway around the areola to maintain nipple viability.

Technique

- Identify affected duct on table by gently squeezing nipple.
- Place lacrimal probe into duct.
- Circumareolar incision with size 15 blade on a Baron's handle.
- Excise affected duct from back of nipple for a length of >2cm. Take a margin of a few mm around the probe (removing the probe with the specimen).
- Mark nipple end with a suture for orientation, and send specimen to pathology.
- Haemostasis.
- Local anaesthetic infiltration.
- Closure with 3-0 Monocryl® (interrupted dermal sutures and a running subcuticular stitch) and Steri-strip™ or glue.
- Same-day discharge.

Total duct excision (Hadfield's operation)

Performed for troublesome nipple discharge from multiple or unidentified ducts or nipple inversion associated with duct ectasia.

Planning/positioning/scar/incision

As for microdochectomy.

Technique

- Circumareolar incision with size 15 blade on a Baron's handle.
- Lift up NAC with skin hooks, and disconnect nipple from major ducts.
- Be careful not to buttonhole the skin when doing this.
- Excise major ducts from back of nipple for a length of >2cm (a square of tissue).
- Mark nipple end with a suture for orientation, and send specimen to pathology.
- Haemostasis: be cautious in the use of diathermy.
- Close defect with 2-0 Vicryl® (undyed).
- A 3-0 Prolene™ purse string under nipple may help reduce/correct nipple inversion (not too tight to maintain blood supply to the nipple).

- Local anaesthetic infiltration.
- Closure with 3-0 Monocryl® (interrupted dermal sutures and a running subcuticular stitch) and Steri-strip™ or glue.
- Same-day discharge.

Complications

See Table 8.1.

Post-operative care

Sutures are dissolvable. Steri-strip™ can be removed at 10 days. Post-operative review can be arranged to discuss results and check wound at 2–3 weeks.

Excision of mammillary fistula

A mammillary fistula (normally at the areolar margin) is the end result of complicated periductal mastitis. It can be excised along with the associated diseased duct passing up to the nipple. However, the risk of recurrence of the fistula is high (up to 50%).

Planning

Mark patient standing up (side, intended scar, and possibly duct involved).

Positioning

Supine with arm by side or abducted to 90°.

Scar/incision

Peri-areolar excising fistula is the best cosmetic way.

Technique

- Place lacrimal probe into fistula.
- Circumareolar incision with size 15 blade on a Baron's handle.
- Excise fistula; clean out any associated abscess cavity and associated duct passing up to the nipple.
- Send specimen to pathology.
- Haemostasis.
- Local anaesthetic infiltration.
- Closure with 3-0 Monocryl® (interrupted dermal sutures and a running subcuticular stitch) and Steri-strip™ or glue. If skin is very indurated, interrupted 3-0 Prolene™ sutures, which need to be removed at 7–10 days, may excite less tissue reaction.
- Same-day discharge.

Table 8.1 Common local complications of nipple surgery to include as part of the consent process

Haematoma	Loss of part of nipple
Infection	Puckering of nipple
Asymmetry	Residual lump
Loss of sensation	Inversion of nipple

Excision of fibroadenoma/benign breast lump

Techniques vary from the use of a vacuum-assisted biopsy device (mammotome) for lesions less than 20mm to a more traditional surgical excision.

Planning

Mark patient standing up (side, intended incision, and position and size of lump).

Positioning

Supine with arm by side.

Scars/incisions

Peri-areolar, inframammary crease, the lateral aspect of the breast, or Langer's Lines.

Technique

- Incise skin, and elevate skin flap towards the lump until you have reached it. Do this in the plane between the subcutaneous fat and the true breast tissue.
- Try to 'fix' the lump with a finger, gently with an Allis forceps, or with a suture.
- Dissect it from the surrounding breast tissue with scalpel, scissors, or diathermy. Common mistake: if there is no clear margin around the lesion you are excising, you have not reached the fibroadenoma yet, go deeper!
- No need for 'margin' of normal breast tissue; can be shelled out intact.
- Ensure haemostasis.
- Local anaesthetic infiltration.
- Closure with 3-0 Monocryl® (interrupted dermal sutures and a running subcuticular stitch) and Steri-strip™ or glue.
- Same-day discharge.

Complications

See Table 8.2.

Post-operative care

Sutures are dissolvable. Steri-strip™ can be removed at 10 days. No routine follow-up is required or a single review to discuss results if there is any concern.

Table 8.2 Common local complications of breast surgery to include as part of the consent process

Haematoma (residual lump felt by patient)	Loss of volume
Infection	Asymmetry
Seroma	Scars
Missed lesion (a palpable area of breast tissue is removed and not the index lesion)	Recurrence

Excision of accessory breast tissue

Normally in the axilla but can be below the breast.

Planning

Mark patient standing up (side, intended incision, and position and size of lump).

Scars/incisions

In skin crease.

Positioning

Supine with arm abducted to 60°.

Technique

- Incise skin, and elevate skin flap beyond the tissue to be excised. Do this in the plane between the subcutaneous fat and the breast tissue.
- Remove accessory breast tissue with scalpel, scissors, or diathermy.
- Ensure haemostasis.
- Local anaesthetic infiltration.
- Closure with 3-0 Monocryl® (interrupted dermal sutures and a running subcuticular stitch) and Steri-strip™ or glue.
- Same-day discharge.

Complications

See Table 8.2.

Post-operative care

Sutures are dissolvable. Steri-strip™ can be removed at 10 days. Follow-up at 6 weeks to assess aesthetic result.

Further reading

Novell JR, Baker D, Goddard N (2013). *Kirk's general surgical operations*, 6e. Elsevier, Philadelphia.

Fitzgerald O'Connor I, Urdang M (2008). *Handbook for surgical cross-cover*. Oxford University Press, Oxford.

Excision of accessory breast tissue

[illegible]

Technique

[illegible]

Further reading

[illegible]

Chapter 9

Gynaecomastia

Overview

Changing nutritional and social habits may explain the reason why there has been a dramatic increase in referrals to breast clinics because of enlargement of the male breast. Gynaecomastia is a benign proliferation of glandular breast tissue, causing enlargement of the male breast. Pseudogynaecomastia has a similar appearance but is due to excess adipose tissue, not glandular tissue. Patients may have a combination of both. Gynaecomastia affects 60% of males at puberty. The incidence increases in advanced age.

Role of primary care

Many gynaecomastia referrals are due to concern about possible significant underlying disease (see Fig. 9.1). GPs should be encouraged to screen out any serious systemic disease prior to referral. In the absence of an obvious clinical underlying cause, GPs should perform:

- Renal, liver, and thyroid function blood tests, and a chest X-ray (CXR). If there is still no clinical underlying cause, perform:
- Endocrine testing: these four markers will screen for any underlying endocrine abnormality:
  - Human chorionic gonadotropin (hCG).
  - Luteinizing hormone (LH).
  - Testosterone.
  - Estradiol.

If any of these blood tests are abnormal, the patient should be referred to an endocrinologist first. When the blood tests are within the normal range, surgical referral is appropriate for patients who would like to discuss treatment options.

History

A standard breast history should be taken. In addition, it is important to record all prescribed drugs. Enquiries must be made of all recreational or illicit drug use, including cannabis, anabolic steroids, and alcohol. It may be tactful to begin this line of enquiry by asking about sporting prowess, gym membership, or even bodybuilding.

Examination

If the blood tests have excluded systemic disease, then the physical examination can be restricted to the breast, axilla, and cervical lymph nodes. Conventional teaching is that the testicles are examined (most commonly in the FRCS exam!). In practice, few contemporary breast surgeons examine the patient's testicles. If the blood tests have excluded systemic illness, then this part of the examination becomes superfluous.

Male breast cancer is rare (7300 new cases a year in the UK). This represents about 1% of all causes of male breast enlargement seen in secondary care. In practice, male breast cancer often has a 'woody' texture on examination, and there is often nipple distortion.

Causes of gynaecomastia

- Idiopathic: the most frequent.
- Physiological: gynaecomastia can occur in neonates, at puberty, and in old age as a result of non-pathological fluctuations in steroid sex hormones.
- Conditions resulting in decreased androgens: primary testicular failure, Klinefelter's syndrome, testicular feminization, bilateral testicular torsion/cryptorchidism, orchitis, renal failure, hyperprolactinaemia.
- Conditions resulting in increased oestrogens: testicular tumours, lung carcinoma, liver disease, thyrotoxicosis, adrenal disease.
- Drug-induced: a large group, particularly in elderly men. Any drug that affects steroid metabolism in the liver might be responsible for gynaecomastia. These include:
  - Hormones: anti-androgens, oestrogen antagonists, treatments particularly associated with carcinoma of the prostate.
  - Cardiovascular: spironolactone, digoxin, ACE inhibitors, amiodarone, verapamil.
  - Gastrointestinal: ranitidine, cimetidine, omeprazole.
  - Others: tricyclic antidepressants, metronidazole, diazepam, metoclopramide, phenytoin, theophylline.
  - Recreational/illicit drugs: cannabis, anabolic steroids, alcohol.

Management

Imaging

Mammography and/or ultrasound (U/S) should only be performed in men with suspicious or unexplained unilateral breast enlargement. U/S can be used to differentiate between true glandular gynaecomastia and fatty pseudogynaecomastia.

Bloods

A biochemical profile should only be performed in men with true gynaecomastia and should include renal and liver function tests. The four blood tests mentioned earlier (see Fig. 9.1) (hCG, LH, testosterone, and estradiol) will highlight any endocrine abnormality. If any of these are abnormal, further discussion with an endocrinologist is required. Ideally, these four blood tests should have been arranged prior to referral.

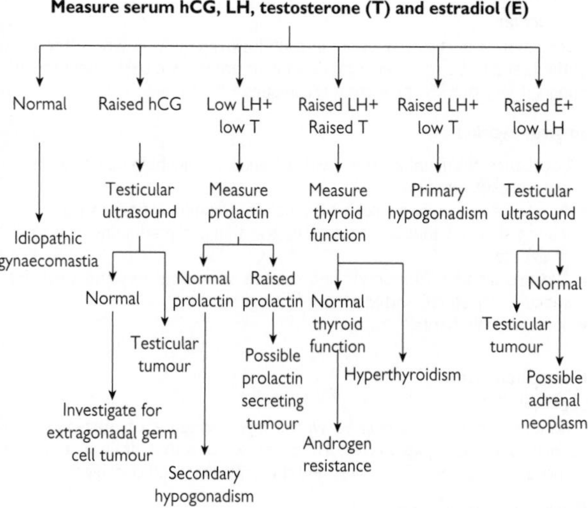

Fig. 9.1 Investigation of a patient with bilateral gynaecomastia.

Excision

For the majority of men, treatment should begin with an explanation of any underlying cause and, if appropriate, a review of prescribed medication. Patients with pubertal gynaecomastia should be reassured, avoiding surgical intervention, if possible. Gynaecomastia has been treated with tamoxifen in the short term, but the evidence base for this is small. Surgery can result in a poor aesthetic outcome and should be approached with caution. Surgical options include those shown in Table 9.1.

Planning

The patient should be standing. Mark the side, inframammary fold, current and desired nipple heights and areola size, intended scars, and extent of resection.

Positioning

Supine with arm by side or abducted to 90°.

Scars/incisions

Peri-areolar, inframammary crease, or at the lateral aspect of the breast.

Technique

Liposuction

Liposuction is particularly useful in pseudogynaecomastia where the bulk of the tissue to be resected is fat. Glandular breasts are best resected with open surgery or U/S liposuction techniques.

Surgical excision

- Local anaesthetic infiltration (with adrenaline, may help haemostasis) pre- or post-excision.
- Aim to avoid nipple necrosis or concavity (dinner plating) by not leaving skin and subcutaneous tissue too thin and graduating to edges of excision.
- Closure with 3-0 Monocryl® (interrupted dermal sutures and a running subcuticular stitch) and Steri-strip™ or glue.
- Same-day discharge.

Complications

See Table 9.2.

As this surgery is associated with a high incidence of post-operative haematoma, many patients return to the ward with a drain *in situ* or a compression garment is applied, and they are observed overnight.

Post-operative care

Sutures are dissolvable. Steri-strip™ can be removed at 7 days. Post-operative review can be arranged to check aesthetic result at 2–3 months.

There are two primary reasons for poor surgical results; in a thin man with primary glandular enlargement, excision can result in a defect that may cause the nipple to sink into the chest wall post-operatively so that the patient exchanges a lump for a concavity.

Conversely, in the patient with fatty enlargement that produces a pseudobreast with ptosis, it is possible to perform liposuction. This may result in there being excessive quantities of redundant skin left behind with an equally poor aesthetic outcome. The complex, and often difficult, decisions required in gynaecomastia surgery demand a multidisciplinary approach with an experienced plastic surgeon.

Patients with gynaecomastia, even when their expectations are realistic, require adequate time and explanation in order to fully understand their options.

Table 9.1 Surgical options for gynaecomastia

Type of surgery	Advantages	Disadvantages
Excision of tissue	Good for removing dense glandular tissue	Scarring and deformity, including nipple scarring to underlying chest wall
Liposuction	Quick. Minimal scarring. Good for pseudogynaecomastia	Cannot always remove dense glandular tissue
Breast/skin reduction	Removes redundant skin in large, ptotic breasts	Extensive, visible scarring

Table 9.2 Common local complications of gynaecomastia surgery to include as part of the consent process

Haematoma	Loss of part of nipple
Infection	Puckering of nipple down to muscle
Asymmetry	Residual lump
Loss of sensation	Inversion of nipple

Chapter 10

Invasive breast carcinoma: pathology and prognosis

Overview

The definition of an invasive breast cancer is one in which the basement membrane of breast ducts and lobules has been breached, allowing the malignant cells to access the surrounding stroma which contains both blood and lymphatic vessels, potentially leading to more widespread dissemination. This contrasts with *in situ* disease in which the basement membrane remains intact, imprisoning the malignant cells (see Chapter 11). For that reason, by definition, *in situ* disease does not metastasize.

Broadly speaking, breast cancers arise from the two major breast unit structures, the ducts and lobules. Therefore, they can be divided into invasive ductal carcinomas which make up about 85% of cancers and invasive lobular carcinomas which account for 10–15% of carcinomas. In addition, there is a small group of special type carcinomas—they arise from specialized parts of these units. They are far less common, tend to be seen in screen-detected tumours, and are associated with a better prognosis.

Infiltrating ductal carcinoma: carcinoma of no special type (NST)

Carcinoma of NST (previously known as ductal carcinoma) is the commonest morphological type (>50% of invasive cancers). Traditionally, these present symptomatically as a hard, irregular, well-defined lump.

Infiltrating lobular carcinoma

Infiltrating lobular carcinoma is the second commonest morphological type (10–15%) of invasive carcinomas. Lobular carcinomas are more commonly multicentric and traditionally associated with a bilateral presentation, although, in reality, the majority affect only one side. The diffuse infiltrating pattern of lobular carcinoma leads to a clinical presentation of diffuse thickening, rather than a defined lump, and, frequently, they are mammographically occult, only being visible on ultrasound. For that reason, patients presenting with an asymmetric thickening and a normal mammogram should have an ultrasound. Lobular carcinomas are often the subject of delay in diagnosis. Because of their diffuse nature, assessment of their size is often best made using ultrasound and MRI. Most MDTs would recommend an MRI in all women considering conservation surgery, following a core biopsy revealing invasive lobular carcinoma. This can change surgical management in up to 28% of cases.

Special types

These are more frequently seen in screening than symptomatic practice.

Tubular carcinoma

Accounts for 15% in screened and 2% in symptomatic. They are seen as a spiculate mass on a mammogram.

Medullary

These account for about 3% of cancers, often associated with BRCA gene mutations. Clinically, they present as a soft lump.

Mucinous carcinomas

These are rare (<1% of invasive carcinomas) and have a well-defined gelatinous appearance. Histologically, tumours consist of epithelial cells within lakes of mucin.

Determining tumour grade

Although it is traditional to histologically type tumours, in practice, an assessment of histological grade is of far more value. The system currently used is that developed by Elston, based on Bloom and Richardson's original scheme. This assesses three aspects of the tumour:

- Tubule formation.
- Nuclear polymorphism.
- Mitotic count.

A numerical scoring system of 1–3 is used for each factor; collation of the three scores gives an overall tumour grade (see Table 10.1).

Other histological factors

There are two other factors, based on basic histopathology, which can contribute to the overall prognosis:

- Lymphovascular invasion and tumour vascularity.
- Extranodal spread in lymph nodes.

Several studies have shown that the presence of tumour cells in vessels, both lymph and blood, is associated with a poorer prognosis for both local and distant recurrence. The density of new vessel growth is also prognostic, although the difficulties in assessing this mean that, in contrast to invasion, it is not routinely reported on pathology reports.

Extranodal spread of tumour in the axilla is, in addition, associated with a poorer overall prognosis.

Table 10.1 The Bloom and Richardson grading system for breast cancers is based upon an additive score of tubule formation, nuclear polymorphism, and mitotic count

Grade	Differentiation	Score
1	Well differentiated	3–5
2	Moderately differentiated	6–7
3	Poorly differentiated	8–9

Molecular factors

Increasingly, molecular factors are being used to assist in prognosis and predict response to treatment. Two particular targets have been identified: the oestrogen receptor and the HER-2 receptor.

Oestrogen receptor status

Since Beatson's observation in 1896 that oophorectomy led to temporary control in some breast cancers, endocrine manipulation has been an essential component of breast cancer management. Laboratory-based technologies can now identify which tumours exhibit strong oestrogen receptor expression. The degree of oestrogen receptor expression in a tumour predicts an individual's response to endocrine therapy. Immunohistochemistry uses monoclonal antibodies to stain nuclear oestrogen receptors. The Allred scoring system collates the two scores for the proportion of positive cells (0–5) and the staining intensity (0–3). A combined score of 0–2 is negative, and a score of 3–8 is considered positive.

Her-2/neu expression

Her1–4 are members of the epidermal growth factor receptor (EGFR) family. The Her-2/neu receptor is expressed on approximately 20% of invasive breast cancers and has a negative impact on patient survival (See Further reading). Immunohistochemistry using monoclonal antibodies to Her-2/neu is used as the primary screen to stain paraffin-embedded tumour tissue. A score of 0–1+ is considered negative, 2+ is equivocal, and a score of 3+ is positive. When a score of 2+ is present, further testing is required using FISH (fluorescent *in situ* hybridization) or D-dish (dual-colour dual-hapten *in-situ* hybridization). FISH is semi-quantitative and directly measures the number of Her-2/neu genes. Patients whose tumours overexpress Her-2 have a poorer prognosis but are candidates for treatment with receptor blockers, such as trastuzumab or lapatanib.

Both these receptors are now used in the routine assessment of breast cancers histologically.

Breast cancer staging

The American Joint Committee on Cancer (AJCC) staging for breast cancer is based upon the TNM (tumour, nodes, metastases) system. The components are shown in Table 10.2.

Table 10.2 AJCC staging for breast cancer

Tumour (T)	
T0	No evidence of primary tumour
Tis	*In situ* carcinoma
T1	<20mm diameter
T2	20–50mm diameter
T3	>50mm diameter
T4	T4a—extension to the chest wall, not including only pectoralis major adherence/invasion T4b—ulceration/ipsilateral satellite nodules/*peau d'orange* T4c—both T4a and T4b T4d—inflammatory carcinoma
Nodes (N) (p—pathology)	
N0	No evidence of lymph node metastases
pN0 (i+)	Malignant cells in regional lymph node(s) <0.2mm, detected by IHC
pN0 (mol+)	Positive molecular findings (RT-PCR), but no regional lymph node metastases detected by IHC or histology
pN1 (mi)	Micrometastases (0.2–2mm) to ipsilateral level I/II axillary lymph node
pN1a	Metastases in 1–3 axillary lymph nodes
pN1b	Metastases to internal mammary lymph nodes, not clinically detected
pN1c	Both pN1a and pN1b
N2	Metastases in ipsilateral level I/II axillary nodes that are fixed or matted, or in clinically detected ipsilateral internal mammary lymph nodes in the absence of involved axillary nodes
N3	Metastases in ipsilateral level III axillary nodes, or in those with clinically involved internal mammary lymph nodes and axillary lymph node metastases, or metastases in the ipsilateral supraclavicular lymph nodes.
Metastases (M)	
cM0(i+)	Deposits of microscopically circulating tumour cells in blood or bone marrow but no clinical or radiological evidence of metastases
M1	Distant detectable metastases >0.2m

Reproduced from AJCC: Breast. In: Edge SB, Byrd DR, Compton CC, eds. AJCC Cancer Staging Manual. 7th ed. New York, NY: Springer, 2010, used with permission of Springer Science and Business Media LLC and the American Joint Committee on Cancer (AJCC).

Prognostic tools in breast cancer

Prognosis in breast cancer depends on time-dependent factors, inherent tumour characteristics, and the response to treatment. Accurate survival estimates and the likely benefit of adjuvant therapy are key pieces of information for patients with early breast cancer. In the UK, the most widely used system is the Nottingham Prognostic Index.

Nottingham Prognostic Index (NPI)

NPI is a validated and reproducible prognostic tool and is based upon three factors:

NPI = [tumour size (cm) x 0.2] + [lymph node stage (1: node negative; 2: 1–3 nodes positive; 3: >3 nodes positive)] + [grade (1–3)]

NPI provides accurate prognostic information and is easy to calculate, based upon three factors that are part of the breast cancer histopathology minimum data set (see Table 10.3). There is a suggestion that, within each prognostic group, screening cancers tend to have a better prognosis.

'Adjuvant! Online'

'Adjuvant! Online' is a decision-making tool that not only gives prognostic information, but also provides projections of the benefit of adjuvant therapy.

Entering a minimum data set of age, co-morbidity, ER status, grade, size, and number of positive nodes will give the clinician a prediction of 10-year survival. 'Adjuvant! Online' will also give a prediction of the absolute benefit of hormonal therapy, chemotherapy, and combined therapy.

Limitations of 'Adjuvant! Online'

'Adjuvant! Online' is based upon the American SEER database; it is for unicentric/unifocal invasive breast carcinomas only and assumes that all patients undergoing breast-conserving surgery will receive adjuvant radiotherapy. At present, 'Adjuvant! Online' does not give prognostic information for Her-2-positive patients, a big disadvantage.

'Predict'

'Predict' is a validated prognostic and treatment benefit tool, based upon UK cancer registry data taken from the Eastern cancer registration and information centre. It has very similar predictive performance to 'Adjuvant! Online'. 'Predict' is also restricted for use on unifocal invasive breast carcinomas and offers prognostic information for Her-2-positive patients and treatment benefit for those offered trastuzumab. 'Predict' includes mode of cancer detection (screen-detected or symptomatic) as one of the input parameters; this is important as stage for stage, screen-detected cancers have a survival advantage over their symptomatic breast cancer counterparts.

Table 10.3 Nottingham Prognostic Index allows us to place patients into a prognostic group with a known and validated 10-year survival

	NPI score	10-year survival (%)
Excellent prognostic group	<2.4	96
Good prognostic group	2.4–<3.4	93
Moderate prognostic group 1	3.4–<4.4	82
Moderate prognostic group 2	4.4–<5.4	75
Poor prognostic group	5.4–<6.4	53
Very poor prognostic group	>6.4	39

Molecular classification of breast cancers and their clinical applications

NPI, 'Adjuvant! Online', and 'Predict' are all predictive/prognostic models that are based on population data and, therefore, do not apply to a specific individual. Several methods are emerging for assessing an individual's future risk of disease and response to treatment, although they are not currently widely used in the UK. These individualized assessment systems include the following.

Oncotype DX

Assesses the expression of 16 cancer genes and five 'housekeeping' (control) genes within an individual's paraffin-embedded cancer tissue. Oncotype DX is only applicable in ER-positive, Her-2-negative tumours and calculates a recurrence score (between 0–100). Patients with a:

- Low recurrence score (1–17): have low risk of cancer recurrence but also respond well to hormonal therapy and have little benefit with chemotherapy.
- High recurrence score (31–100): have a high risk of recurrence and gain a great benefit from chemotherapy.
- For patients with a moderate recurrence score (18–30), it is unclear whether there is a benefit from chemotherapy. The TAILORx ((Trial Assigning Individualized Options for Treatment (Rx)) trial has been designed to help define the role of chemotherapy, particularly in patients with a moderate recurrence score.
- NICE is likely to approve the use of Oncotype DX for Intermediate risk (as per NPI/Predict), ER positive, node negative patients. Results of the initial consultation are in Further reading.

Mammaprint

Mammaprint analyses a gene signature of 70 breast cancer-related genes and places patients in a high- or low-risk recurrence group. Access to the test may be limited, as the analysis must be performed on fresh/frozen tissue in the Netherlands. Mammaprint is able to define the benefit of adjuvant chemotherapy for a given patient's cancer. Mammaprint can be used for cancers up to 5cm in size, ER-positive or -negative, and node-positive or -negative. Mammaprint is costly (>£2,500) and has not yet been validated on a UK population.

Further reading

Mann RM, Hoogeveen, YL, Blickman JG, Boetes C (2008). MRI compared to conventional diagnostic work-up in the detection and evaluation of invasive lobular carcinoma of the breast: a review of existing literature. *Breast Cancer Res Treat* **107**, 1–14.

Slamon DJ, Clark GM, Wong SG, *et al.* (1987). Human breast cancer: correlation of relapse and survival with amplification of the Her-2/neu oncogene *Science* **235**, 177–82.

Tovey S, Brown S, Doughty J, Mallon E (2009). Poor survival outcomes in Her-2 positive patients with low-grade, node negative tumours. *Br J Cancer* **100**, 680–3.

Moja L, Tagliabue L, Balduzzi S, *et al.* (2012). Trastuzumab containing regimens for early breast cancer. *Cochrane Database Syst Rev* **4**, CD006243.

Barr LC, Baum M (1992). Time to abandon TNM staging of breast cancer. *Lancet* **339**, 915–17.

Adjuvant! Online. Available at: ☞ http://www.adjuvantonline.com

The PREDICT tool. Available at: ☞ http://www.predict.nhs.uk

Gene expression profiling and expanded immunohistochemistry tests to guide the use of adjuvant chemotherapy in early breast cancer management - MammaPrint, Oncotype DX, IHC4 and Mammostrat: diagnostics consultation document 3 (PDF version) available at: ☞ http://guidance.nice.org.uk/DT/4/Consultation3/DraftGuidance/pdf/English

Further reading

Chapter 11

Non-invasive breast disease: DCIS, lobular pathologies, and hyperplasias

Overview

The introduction of the NHS Breast Screening Programme has resulted in a large increase in the proportion of cases of pre-malignant breast disease. Improved pathological methods also detect non-invasive breast disease in a significant number of patients.

Definition

- Also known as *in situ* breast disease.
- Malignant cells remain within ducts/lobules (see Fig. 11.1).
- Do NOT invade the basement membrane.

Types

- Atypical ductal hyperplasia (ADH).
- Ductal carcinoma *in situ* (DCIS).
- Atypical lobular hyperplasia (ALH).
- Lobular carcinoma *in situ* (LCIS) (can be known as lobular *in situ* neoplasia [LIN]).

Non-invasive breast pathologies are a spectrum of disease. Atypical ductal hyperplasia has the same pathological features as DCIS, but usually it is only an increase in the quantity seen on pathology that will upgrade the diagnosis to DCIS. Due to the lack of longitudinal studies of DCIS, the natural history of low- and intermediate-grade DCIS is uncertain. High-grade DCIS will develop into an invasive cancer; the time lag before this occurs, however, is also uncertain. Much of the debate about the benefit of the NHSBSP revolves around 'overdiagnosis' of breast cancers; the majority of these overdiagnoses are likely to be non-invasive breast cancers, the future prognosis of which we are currently unable to predict.

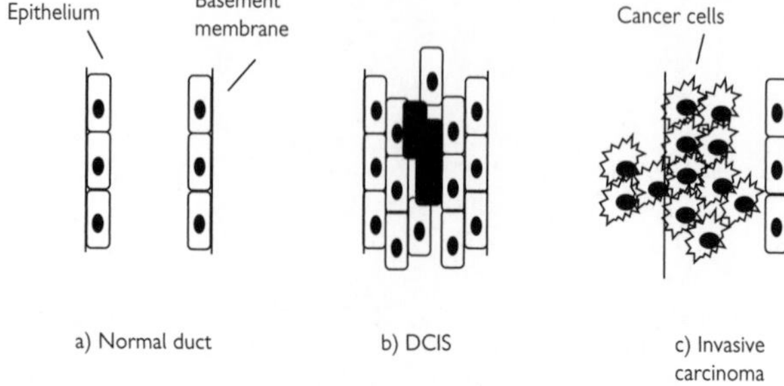

Fig. 11.1 Carcinoma sequence for breast cancer. a) Normal duct with epithelial lining. b) DCIS. Tumour has grown within the duct but does not penetrate the basement membrane. Tumour cells in the centre lose vascular supply (black cells in figure), become necrotic, and calcify. Micro-calcification is visible on mammography. c) Invasive carcinoma—tumour cells have grown and invaded into the lumen and out through the duct wall and basement membrane. They now have an increased potential to metastasize.

Atypical ductal hyperplasia

- Abnormal cells within breast ducts.
- Involves <2 ducts or is <2–3mm in size.
- Possible precursor to low-grade DCIS.

Diagnosis

- Visible on mammograms if associated with micro-calcification.
- May be incidental finding after excision biopsy.

Prognosis

- 25% risk of developing invasive disease.
- Risk increased in presence of DCIS.

Treatment

- If diagnosed on core biopsy, requires excision biopsy, as it is often adjacent to *in situ* or invasive cancer.
- If incidental finding in association with invasive disease, no further treatment is necessary.

Follow-up

- Regular mammographic surveillance should be discussed.
- High-risk patients may benefit from chemoprevention (not licensed in UK).

Ductal carcinoma *in situ*

- Accounts for ~20% of screen-detected breast tumours in UK.
- Abnormal proliferation of cells within milk ducts.
- 90% of cases are impalpable and asymptomatic.
- 10% of cases are associated with symptoms—mass, nipple discharge, Paget's disease.

Diagnosis

- 70–80% of cases associated with micro-calcification—visible on mammograms (see Fig. 11.1).
- As impalpable, requires stereotactic-guided biopsy.
- Marker clip should be inserted at time of biopsy.
- Presence of micro-calcifications should be confirmed in cores.

Pathology

- Graded by cytological features: low, intermediate, and high grade (observer-dependent).
- Low/intermediate grade may arise from ADH/LIN due to loss of 16q.
- High grade exhibits 17p loss and has no known precursor.
- High-grade DCIS associated with increased Her-2 and decreased ER expression.
- Architectural subtypes: papillary, micropapillary, solid, comedo, cribriform.
- Majority of screen-detected DCIS is high-grade (~60%).

Prognosis

- Risk of developing invasive breast cancer unknown.
- Up to 33% future breast cancer risk for low-grade DCIS.

Treatment

- In general, if <4cm area of DCIS: image-guided wide local excision.
- Up to 30% of cases may require re-excision (NICE guidelines, 2mm margin).
- >4cm or multifocal disease: mastectomy ± reconstruction.
- Axillary surgery is not currently recommended for simple cases of DCIS alone.
- Sentinel node biopsy is indicated if performing a mastectomy for DCIS or if there is an associated mass.

Recurrence risk

- Following breast-conserving surgery only, 25% risk of recurrent disease (either DCIS or invasive).
- Important risk factors: <1mm margins, high grade, comedo necrosis, poorly differentiated, age <40 years.
- USC/Van Nuys prognostic index scores, DCIS grade, margin status, tumour size, and patient age to predict local recurrence and suggest treatment options (see Table 11.1). It is rarely used in clinical practice but does demonstrate risk factors associated with local recurrence.

Adjuvant treatment

- Radiotherapy: reduces ipsilateral recurrence but no survival advantage. Recommended for high-grade DCIS.
- Endocrine therapy: reduces local recurrence in ER-positive cases and may reduce contralateral cancer incidence. Tamoxifen recommended if <50 years. Current IBIS II trial comparing tamoxifen and aromatase inhibitor.

Follow-up

- Following breast-conserving surgery, annual mammography is recommended.

Table 11.1 USC/Van Nuys prognostic index

Score	**1**	**2**	**3**
DCIS grade	Low/int, no necrosis	Low/int, with necrosis	High ± necrosis
Margin (mm)	>10	1–9	<1
Size (mm)	<15	16–40	>41
Age (y)	>61	40–60	<39
Score	**Local recurrence risk**	**Suggested treatment**	**Score**
4–6	1%	Local excision, no radiotherapy	4–6
7–9	20%	Local excision and radiotherapy	7–9
10–12	50%	Mastectomy	10–12

Lobular intraepithelial neoplasia (LIN)

- Includes atypical lobular hyperplasia (ALH) (part of lobule affected) and LCIS (whole lobule affected).
- Not a pre-malignant condition, but a marker of breast cancer risk.
- Abnormal cells within breast lobules.

Diagnosis

- 90% of cases detected in pre-menopausal women.
- Not usually visible on mammograms.
- Incidental finding on biopsy or surgical excision.
- 50% have multifocal disease.
- 30% have bilateral disease.
- 50% have a family history of breast cancer.

Prognosis

- 25% risk of developing invasive disease.
- Risk increased if family history of breast cancer and in presence of ADH or DCIS.
- Pleomorphic phenotype may be associated with poorer prognosis.

Treatment

- If diagnosed on core biopsy, requires excision biopsy.
- If incidental finding in association with invasive disease, no further treatment is necessary.
- No indication for radiotherapy or chemotherapy.

Follow-up

- Increased surveillance (MRI may be optimal, as disease not visible on mammograms).
- Chemoprevention with tamoxifen or raloxifene (not currently licensed in the UK).
- Young or high-risk patients may opt for risk-reducing mastectomy.

Further reading

Silverstein MJ, Buchanan C (2003). Ductal carcinoma *in situ:* USC/Van Nuys Prognostic Index and the impact of margin status. *Breast* **12**, 457–71.

Julien JP, Bijker N, Fentiman IS, *et al.* (2000). Radiotherapy in breast-conserving treatment for ductal carcinoma *in situ:* first results of the EORTC randomised phase III trial 10853. EORTC Breast Cancer Cooperative Group and EORTC Radiotherapy Group. *Lancet* **355**, 528–33.

Fisher ER, Dignam J, Tan-Chiu E, *et al.* (1999). Pathologic findings from the National Surgical Adjuvant Breast Project (NSABP) eight-year update of Protocol B-17: intraductal carcinoma. *Cancer* **86**, 429–38.

Fisher B, Dignam J, Wolmark N, *et al.* (1999). Tamoxifen in treatment of intraductal breast cancer: National Surgical Adjuvant Breast and Bowel Project B-24 randomised controlled trial. *Lancet* **353**, 1993–2000.

Houghton J, George WD, Cuzick J, *et al.* (2003). Radiotherapy and tamoxifen in women with completely excised ductal carcinoma *in situ* of the breast in the UK, Australia, and New Zealand: randomized controlled trial. *Lancet* **362**, 95–102.

Chapter 12

Basic surgery for breast cancer and the management of margins

Surgical considerations

The results of the triple assessment should be discussed with the patient by the operating surgeon, accompanied by a breast care nurse (BCN). It is important that all the relevant treatment options agreed by the MDT are explained, and the patient should be given time to make a fully informed choice about their treatment. Information leaflets should be provided along with a contact number for the BCN.

Preoperative assessment

All patients should undergo formal preoperative assessment prior to their definitive surgery. The aim is to identify any significant co-morbidities and to address any concerns which the patient may have about their operation. If there is any doubt about the fitness of the patient for a particular procedure, it should be discussed with the anaesthetist doing the case prior to admission.

Consent for the operation should be sought by a member of the surgical team who is capable of performing the procedure and should include all significant and common risks associated with the procedure.

Surgical options

Each patient's body shape is unique, and the challenge is to match sound oncological excision with the best aesthetic outcome. In addition, the patient's general health and psychological make-up may modify the surgical options. In general, once more than 20% of the breast has been excised, a significant defect will be created. In practice, this means that, for most patients, the options are:

- Wide local excision.
- Wide local excision and therapeutic mammoplasty.
- Mastectomy.
- Mastectomy and reconstruction.

Tumours <2cm in diameter, or those with a favourable tumour-to-breast volume ratio, are suitable for wide local excision (WLE). Tumours involving the nipple may require mastectomy, although central WLE is also acceptable, depending on patient choice. All WLE cases for invasive cancer require a course of post-operative radiotherapy. The possible need for re-excision to obtain clear margins should be discussed, particularly if non-invasive disease has been found to be mixed with invasive on biopsy.

Mastectomy is usually required for those cancers where the tumour-to-breast volume ratio is adverse. In these cases, the options for reconstruction need to be considered. Oncoplastic techniques and specific procedures are discussed in Chapters 18 and 19, but the oncological principles detailed here are still applicable.

In invasive cancer, preoperative ultrasound and biopsy of axillary nodes will have indicated whether there is axillary disease present. If no abnormal lymph nodes are detected in cases of invasive cancer, a sentinel lymph node biopsy (SLNB) is performed. Involved axillary lymph nodes mandate an axillary lymph node clearance (ANC). In DCIS which is to be managed by WLE, there is no indication for axillary surgery. The exception to this is when imaging is highly suggestive of a focus of invasive disease (e.g. visible mass on ultrasound or mammography, larger area of disease, high-grade disease); in this situation, a sentinel node biopsy at the time of WLE can be offered. If mastectomy is required for extensive or multifocal DCIS, a sentinel node biopsy is appropriate.

Management of margins

There are no high-quality randomized data to determine what an acceptable post-operative margin is that does not require further tissue excision (see Further reading). Principles in assessing margin adequacy include:

- Increasing the width of an acceptable post-operative pathological margin around a tumour is weakly associated with lower odds of local recurrence.
- Cavity shaves (taking radial cavity shaves at the time of cancer surgery) can decrease the need for re-excision surgery.
- A radial margin involved with tumour should be re-excised. Any margin around an invasive cancer may be adequate; a larger margin may be preferable in DCIS.
- Anterior/posterior margins involved with tumour may not need re-excision, as often these cannot be surgically improved upon. Adjuvant radiotherapy has a role in many of these patients to decrease the risk of local recurrence.
- Individual units must know their local recurrence rate, as this determines if their margin management is of an adequate standard. Local policy will dictate margin size.

Breast-conserving surgery

Indications

- Patient choice.
- Small tumour-to-breast volume.

In practice, most early breast cancers, particularly screen-detected cancers up to 2cm in size, are suitable for conservation. However, a patient with E cup size breasts and a 4cm tumour may be suitable for conservation.

Preoperative preparation

- Impalpable tumours require image-guided localization.
- Methods include wire placement, ultrasound marking, or radioguided occult lesion localization (ROLL).
- Palpable tumours should be marked preoperatively by the surgeon.
- If, at the time of marking, there is doubt in the surgeon's mind about location of the tumour, even in symptomatic cases, preoperative image guidance is appropriate.
- It is courteous to confirm the timing of localization with the radiologist who will also have a busy schedule.

Simple mastectomy

Indications

- Locally advanced tumours, including inflammatory cancers.
- Large tumour-to-breast volume ratio.
- Central tumours involving nipple, although this is not mandatory.
- Recurrent breast cancer.
- Multifocal or widespread DCIS.

Sentinel lymph node biopsy

Indications

- In invasive cancer when the preoperative ultrasound assessment ± FNA has shown the axillary nodes to be apparently normal.
- When performing mastectomy for DCIS.
- Prior to immediate breast reconstruction in patients at risk of needing adjuvant radiotherapy (see Chapter 19).
- Sentinel node biopsy does carry a minimal risk of arm morbidity, including lymphoedema, a stiff arm, and numbness (see Further reading).

Axillary lymph node clearance

Indications

- Involved axillary lymph nodes in the presence of invasive disease on preoperative ultrasound and biopsy.
- Positive SLNB (this is the subject of much current debate—see Box 12.1 and Further reading).
- Loco-regional disease recurrence.

Box 12.1 Current opinion—management of a positive sentinel node biopsy

- Options for axillary treatment following a positive sentinel node biopsy are:
  - Axillary clearance.
  - Axillary radiotherapy.
  - Whole breast radiotherapy (WBRT)—following breast conservation surgery.
- This is a fast-moving area of contention; guidance, the evidence base, and practice are rapidly changing.
- Historically, all patients received axillary clearance following the identification of a positive sentinel node.
- Arguments in favour of axillary clearance:
  - Surgery removes all involved nodes and, therefore, reduces burden of disease.
  - It reduces the risk of axillary recurrent disease.
  - It generally avoids the need for axillary radiotherapy.
  - Some patients may be at higher risk of axillary recurrent disease and, therefore, show a survival advantage following ANC. We are, as yet, unable to identify this group preoperatively.
  - ANC accurately stages the axilla and can change adjuvant treatment. Those with four, or more, involved nodes will be given chest wall, axillary, and supraclavicular radiotherapy.
- Arguments against routine axillary clearance following identification of a positive sentinel node:
  - The majority of patients undergoing ANC will have no further positive nodes identified. The operation is, therefore, overtreatment for the majority.
  - If no ANC is performed, local recurrence after a positive SNB is rare.
  - ANC does not confer a survival advantage following SNB in post-menopausal women requiring whole breast irradiation (WBRT).
  - Radiation to the axilla reduces the risk of local recurrence and reduces the risk of lymphoedema compared to ANC, but it does increase the incidence of a stiff arm.

Currently, an approach for SNB-positive women may be:

- Pre-menopausal: little available evidence. Likely to be a higher risk group—ANC.
- Post-menopausal women:
  - Following WLE: low-risk T1/T2 tumours—WBRT.
  - Following WLE: high-risk tumours (T3/4, Her-2-positive)—ANC.
  - Following mastectomy—ANC.

Further reading

Mansel RE, Fallowfield L, Kissin M, *et al.* (2006). Randomized multicenter trial of sentinel node biopsy versus standard axillary treatment in operable breast cancer: the ALMANAC. *J Natl Cancer Inst* **98**, 599–609.

Giuliano AE, Hunt KK, Ballman KV, *et al.* (2011). Axillary dissection vs no axillary dissection in women with invasive breast cancer and sentinel node metastasis: a randomized clinical trial. *JAMA* **305**, 569–75.

Setton J, Cody H, Tan L, *et al.* (2012). Radiation field design and regional control in sentinel lymph node-positive breast cancer patients with omission of axillary dissection. *Cancer* **118**, 1994–2003.

Giuliano AE, Morrow M, Duggal S, Julian TB (2012). Should ACOSOG Z0011 change practice with respect to axillary lymph node dissection for a positive sentinel lymph node biopsy in breast cancer? *Clin Exp Metastasis* **29**, 687–92.

Houssami N, Macaskill P, Marinovich M, *et al.* (2010). Meta-analysis of the impact of surgical margins on local recurrence in women with early –stage invasive breast cancer treated with breast-conserving surgery. *Eur J Cancer* **46**, 3219–32.

Morrow M, Harris J, Schnitt S (2012). Surgical margins in lumpectomy for breast cancer—bigger is not better. *N Engl J Med* **367**, 79–82.

Chapter 13

Adjuvant therapy

Benefits of adjuvant therapy

The use of adjuvant therapy following surgery in patients with breast cancer has been a significant factor in the reduction in breast cancer mortality seen in Western countries over the last 20 years. The aim of adjuvant therapy is to prevent or delay recurrence by treating residual micrometastatic disease with both systemic and local treatments following surgery. There are four modalities of adjuvant therapy commonly used:

- Radiotherapy (local treatment).
- Hormone manipulation (systemic treatment).
- Chemotherapy (systemic treatment).
- Biological modifiers (systemic treatment).

Radiotherapy

The prime role of radiotherapy (DXT) is in treating residual disease in the breast and chest wall and sometimes the axilla. Its use after breast conservation significantly reduces local recurrence.

The common situations in which radiotherapy is employed are:

- Following wide local excision (WLE) for invasive cancer, almost invariably.
- Following wide local excision for some cases of DCIS.
- Following mastectomy in high-risk cases.
- Occasionally to the axilla following a positive axillary sampling or SNB.

The commonest indication is following a WLE for invasive cancer once the margins are clear. In these circumstances, whole breast radiotherapy is the rule, and not employing it would be difficult to justify, except in rare circumstances. Precise protocols may vary between centres, but the usual dose is 20Gy spread over 3 weeks. The dose is delivered to the whole breast, often with a tumour bed boost. The IMPORT trial is currently investigating more tumour bed-targeted therapy which is why the insertion of titanium clips at surgery is now becoming standard protocol in some centres in order to facilitate targeting.

Radiotherapy following WLE for DCIS is more controversial and more subject to local variations in practice. Whilst some regard it as a substitute for inadequate surgery, other centres employ it routinely for all but very small, areas of low-grade DCIS, using prognostic factors as a guide. It is not suitable for widespread multifocal disease.

Use after mastectomy to the chest wall, axilla, and supraclavicular regions is frequently recommended for:

- Large tumours (>5cm).
- Close or involved margins.
- 4+ node-positive tumours.
- Lymphovascular invasion.

The PRIME study is currently comparing the value of radiotherapy in apparently less aggressive tumours following mastectomy with the more established indication (see Further reading).

Axillary radiotherapy is the most controversial. It is contraindicated in patients who have undergone axillary node clearance. However, it has been advocated for patients who have undergone an axillary node sampling who are found to have involved nodes (see Chapter 12). With the introduction of sentinel node biopsy, this procedure is becoming less common; however, the AMAROS study is assessing the benefits of radiotherapy, as opposed to salvage clearance, for patients who have involved sentinel nodes. This trial shows equivalence in cancer outcomes between the two cohorts.

Hormonal manipulation

The use of hormonal manipulation in breast cancer dates back to the late 19th century when Beatson observed the beneficial effects of oophorectomy in locally advanced breast cancer. Despite Beatson's observation, adjuvant endocrine therapy only became widespread with the introduction of tamoxifen in the 1980s. Clinical trials showed a clear survival benefit for those patients receiving tamoxifen. It took some years for clinicians to fully recognize that hormonal therapy was not indicated in women whose tumours are ER-negative.

The mechanisms available for hormone manipulation now are:

- Hormone blockade at cellular level.
- Pharmacological disruption of hormone production.
- Oophorectomy.

As a therapy, it is only of benefit and its use is confined to oestrogen receptor-positive tumours.

Hormone blockade

The classic drug associated with this was tamoxifen, which, for many years, was the mainstay of hormonal adjuvant treatment. It had both oestrogen agonist and antagonist properties. In bone, it behaved as an oestrogen whereas, in the breast, its properties were antagonistic. It remains in common use for pre-menopausal women and has recently been replaced in post-menopausal women by aromatase inhibitors.

Pharmacological disruption of hormone production

Despite its effects when first used, it was recognized that some patients seemed resistant to blockade with tamoxifen, which led to a search for means of blocking oestrogen production. The prime sources of oestrogen are the ovaries in pre-menopausal women and the adrenals and peripheral fat in post-menopausal women. Originally, oophorectomy, adrenalectomy, and hypophysectomy were used as therapeutic manoeuvres in the treatment of recurrence. These were obviously very invasive and not ideal as adjuvant treatment. It was recognized that two mechanisms could be targeted pharmacologically to disrupt production. In post-menopausal women, most oestrogen comes from peripheral aromatization of testosterone, which can now be blocked using a new generation of aromatase inhibitors which block this step. Three drugs are in common use: anastrozole, exemestane, and letrozole. Of these, the ATAC study demonstrated a significant improvement in disease-free interval with the use of anastrozole compared to tamoxifen, and similar advantages were seen in the Big 1-98 study with letrozole. Consequently, these two drugs are used, according to local preference, as the first-line hormone manipulation in post-menopausal ER-positive patients. Exemestane has been used as a cross-over drug; patients who have already had 2 years of treatment with tamoxifen are swapped over for a further 3 years of exemestane treatment.

In pre-menopausal women, oestrogen comes from the ovary so that aromatase inhibitors confer no benefit, as they do not block this ovarian oestrogen production. Tamoxifen directly blocks oestrogen receptors in the cancer cell, therefore, blocking all oestrogen stimulation, no matter what the site of production. Tamoxifen is the first-line drug in pre-menopausal women. Alternatively, chemical or surgical oophorectomy can be used as an adjuvant hormonal treatment. Goserelin is a gonadotropin-releasing hormone (GnRH) which, when given at a continuous dose, inhibits both oestrogen and testosterone production. It is given as a depot injection every 3 months for 2 years and abolishes ovarian oestrogen production. Its great advantage over surgical oophorectomy is that it is potentially reversible. In practice, relatively few tumours in pre-menopausal women are receptor-positive so that hormone manipulation in the pre-menopausal is less common. When it is used, a frequent regimen is goserelin for 2 years (in combination with 6 months of chemotherapy), followed by tamoxifen.

Chemotherapy

Not all patients benefit from chemotherapy in the adjuvant setting, with the benefit depending on the individual patient's risk. Data on these benefits are available from the Early Breast Cancer Trials Collaborative Group (EBCTCG) which reviews and updates results from relevant randomized trials every 5 years. A total of 28,000 patients have been entered into studies looking at adjuvant chemotherapy vs no chemotherapy, and overall there is a 10% survival benefit seen at 15 years for patients receiving chemotherapy. Younger women (<50 years) have a greater reduction in their risk of recurrence with chemotherapy than women between 50 and 70 years (30% vs 12%). Patients with both ER-positive and -negative tumours gain a similar proportional benefit with chemotherapy; however, the absolute gain is greater in patients with ER-poor tumours.

Indications for adjuvant chemotherapy

The decision to recommend adjuvant chemotherapy is made with the patient by discussing the potential benefits of treatment and weighing these against the treatment-related toxicities. Thus, accurate assessment of an individual's risk of loco-regional recurrence and mortality is important in order to gauge the true risk/benefit ratio. Prognostic tools have been developed to give an estimation of breast cancer mortality, based on combinations of known prognostic factors (see Chapter 10), such as:

- Tumour size.
- Histological grade.
- Nodal involvement.
- Oestrogen/progesterone receptor status.
- Patient age.
- Her-2/neu status (see Biological modifiers in this chapter).
- Lymphovascular invasion.

A number of groups have produced consensus guidelines identifying risk groups and recommending treatment strategies. The European International Consensus Panel Guidelines (2005) are summarized (see Table 13.1 and Further reading):

Risk category

Low risk

Node-negative and:

- Tumour <2cm, and
- Grade 1, and
- No lymphovascular invasion, and
- Her2 gene not overexpressed,
- Age >35 years.

Intermediate risk

Node-negative and at least one of:

- Tumour >2cm, or
- Grade 2–3, or
- Presence of lymphovascular invasion, or
- Her-2 gene overexpressed, or
- Age <35 years,
- Node-positive (1–3) and Her-2 gene not overexpressed.

High risk

- Node-positive (1–3 nodes) and Her-2 overexpressed.
- Node-positive (4, or more, involved nodes).

In addition to this approach, the Nottingham Prognostic Index (NPI) can be used to stratify patients according to risk of death. More recently, computer-generated models, such as Adjuvant! Online and 'Predict', have been used to compare the relative benefits of the various adjuvant regimes as an aid to decision-making (see Prognostic tools in breast cancer in Chapter 10).

Table 13.1 Summary of the European guidelines for prescribing adjuvant treatment

Risk category	Endocrine responsive	Endocrine non-responsive
Low	ET or nil	Nil
Intermediate	ET or CT + ET	CT
High	CT + ET	CT

ET, endocrine therapy; CT, chemotherapy.

Chemotherapy regimens

A large number of regimens have been used that can be divided broadly into those containing anthracyclines and those that do not. Older regimens commonly did not include anthracyclines, which have been shown to confer a 5% survival advantage at 10 years. Treatment is commonly given three weekly for 4–6 months. Anthracyclines are associated with both a dose-dependent and idiosyncratic risk of cardiac impairment.

Taxane-containing regimes

Multiple studies have looked at the benefit of adding a taxane to anthracycline-based regimes. There is significant heterogeneity between the trials in terms of regimens used, duration of treatment, and patient population studied. Although the addition of a taxane has not shown a survival benefit in all trials, there is evidence of benefit, particularly in patients with node-positive disease, and taxane therapy should be considered for this patient group (see Further reading).

Side effects of chemotherapy

Although the treatment of chemotherapy-related toxicities has improved, both potential acute and long-term side effects need to be discussed with the patient and form part of the decision-making process (see Following systemic therapies in Chapter 14).

- Nausea and vomiting.
- Sore mouth—ulcers/infection.
- Fatigue.
- Hair loss.
- Menopausal symptoms and premature menopause.
- Sexual difficulties.
- Diarrhoea.
- Neutropenia.
- Bleeding.
- Nail disorders.
- Limb oedema.
- Weight loss/gain.
- Depression/anxiety.
- Cardiac impairment (especially with anthracyclines).
- Infections.

Biological modifiers: Her-2/neu and adjuvant trastuzumab (Herceptin®)

Her-2/neu (human epidermal growth factor receptor 2) is a cell surface tyrosine kinase receptor-like molecule, which is involved in signal transduction pathways regulating cell growth and differentiation. Eighteen to 20% of breast cancers overexpress this protein, and this overexpression is also associated with a poorer prognosis. Tumours are classified as overexpressing Her-2 if they score 3+ on immunohistochemical staining or are positive on fluorescent *in situ* hybridization (FISH).

Trastuzumab is a humanized murine monoclonal antibody to the Her-2/neu protein. A number of large US and multinational trials have looked at the use of trastuzumab in the adjuvant setting. Patients enrolled in these studies were either node-positive or high-risk node-negative, and all received adjuvant chemotherapy. After a short follow-up, the results of these studies have shown a similar significant improvement in both disease-free and overall survival. Treatment with trastuzumab does carry a risk of cardiac toxicity, with up to 4% risk of a significant reduction in left ventricular function. This has been seen with a follow-up of 2–3 years, and the long-term effects on the heart are unknown. Lapatinib is an oral tyrosine kinase inhibitor that has not yet been approved by NICE outside the context of clinical trials. Lapatinib shows promise in combination with trastuzumab and in the context of metastatic disease (see Further reading).

Further advances

With greater understanding of the molecular processes involved in cancer, it is proving possible to pinpoint specific molecules with pivotal functions in cell growth and division which can be targeted pharmacologically. As yet, many of these drugs are in early development, although some are making their way through to early phase 1 trials. If successful, it is likely that the next 10 years will see a major revolution in much more personalized and targeted therapy for breast cancer that might even render surgery redundant!

Further reading

Goldhirsch A, Wood WC, Coates AS, *et al.* (2011). Strategies for subtypes—dealing with the diversity of breast cancer: highlights of the St. Gallen International Expert Consensus on the Primary Therapy of Early Breast Cancer 2011. *Ann Oncol* **22**, 1736–47.

Goldhirsch A, Glick JH, Gelber RD, *et al.* (2005). Meeting highlights: international expert consensus on the primary therapy of early breast cancer 2005. *Ann Oncol* **16**, 1569–83.

Prescott RJ, Kunkler IH, Williams LJ, *et al.* (2007). A randomised controlled trial of post-operative radiotherapy following breast-conserving surgery in a minimum-risk older population. The PRIME trial. *Health Technol Assess* **11**, 1–149.

Cuzick J, Sestak I, Baum M, *et al.* (2010). Effect of anastrozole and tamoxifen as adjuvant treatment for early stage breast cancer: 10 year analysis of the ATAC trial. *Lancet Oncol* **11**, 1135–41.

Coates AS, Keshaviah A, Thurlimann B, *et al.* (2007). Five years of letrozole compared with tamoxifen as initial adjuvant therapy for postmenopausal women with endocrine responsive early breast cancer: update of study BIG 1-98. *J Clin Oncol* **25**, 486–92.

Early Breast Cancer Trials Collaborative Group (EBCTCG) (2005). Effects of chemotherapy and hormonal therapy for early breast cancer on recurrence and 15-year survival: an overview of the randomized trials. *Lancet* **365**, 1687–717.

Early Breast Cancer Trials Collaborative Group (EBCTCG) (2011). Effect of radiotherapy after breast-conserving surgery on 10 year recurrence and 15-year breast cancer death: meta-analysis of individual patient data for 10,801 women in 17 randomised trails. *Lancet* **378**, 1707–16.

Early Breast Cancer Trials Collaborative Group (EBCTCG) (2012). Comparisons between different polychemotherapy regimens for early breast cancer: meta-analysis of long-term outcome among 100,000 women in 123 randomised trials. *Lancet* **379**, 432–44.

Blackwell KL, Burstein HJ, Storniolo AM, *et al.* (2010). Randomized study of lapatinib alone or in combination with trastuzumab in women with ErbB2-positive, trastuzumab-refractory metastatic breast cancer. *J Clin Oncol* **28**, 1124–30.

The ALTTO trial. Available at: http://www.alttotrials.com

Chapter 14

Treatment-induced complications

Following surgery

Post-operative complications can be split into those specific to the operation concerned and the general complications of surgery. Only the former will be covered in any detail here.

Risk factors for complications

- Smoking.
- Obesity.
- Diabetes.
- Prior breast or chest wall radiotherapy.
- Connective tissue disorders.

Immediate complications

Haemorrhage/excessive blood in drains. Assess need for circulatory support, and have blood available if bleeding copiously. Ensure good intravenous (IV) access, and arrange urgent return to theatre to stop the bleeding. Blood does not need to be cross-matched prior to a mastectomy.

Early complications (within 24 hours)

- Haematoma: bruising or discoloration of the skin over a tense swollen wound. A result of reactionary haemorrhage. Small bleeding vessels thrombose, as the pressure from the haematoma rises, but, if left untreated, a haematoma will be a source of discomfort and potential infection and will impede wound healing. Once the patient is adequately resuscitated, FBC, clotting, and G&S should be obtained, and the patient should return to theatre for evacuation of haematoma and to try and identify the bleeding point. In general, it is better to evacuate a haematoma than to hope it will 'resolve' with time.

Of note: excessive bleeding is often associated with minimal blood in the drains (as the drains clot off). If you even think about the need for evacuation, DO IT! Ensure this strategy is clearly handed over to any subsequent shifts.

- Necrosis/breakdown of wound edges: a small area of simple wound breakdown can be cleaned up and occasionally re-sutured if the edges are healthy.

Following reconstructive or plastic surgery

- The viability of skin flaps, the nipple, and the transposed flaps can all be threatened by undue pressure on the flap, venous congestion, hypotension, or arterial insufficiency. These complications are the highest risk of modern oncoplastic surgery; as such, wards and units carrying out this type of surgery need good training in recognizing potential problems. There need to be well-established protocols for the post-operative care of patients. When complications do occur, it is important to enlist the help of other specialists, such as wound care nurses and plastic surgeons.

- Accurate handover of the status of free flaps should occur at the end of each shift. This ensures awareness of the patients requiring careful observation overnight and continuity of care.
- Myocutaneous flap failure: a cold flap (white with arterial insufficiency/ purple with venous congestion) with poor capillary return is a cause for alarm. Consider urgent return to theatre to avoid flap loss. Free flaps are less robust than pedicled (LD or TRAM) flaps.
- Skin flap necrosis: this occurs with a thin or devascularized mastectomy flap, more commonly on the side of an axillary clearance where the lateral blood supply to the breast has been interrupted. Exclude haematoma; optimize perfusion, and excise frankly necrotic skin before secondary repair or inserting a skin graft or flap to close any defect.
- Nipple congestion/discoloration: may need some sutures removed or leeches applied to decrease tension. Discuss with a senior first.
- Sloughing of abdominal wounds or umbilical necrosis after TRAM/ DIEP, secondary to extensive tissue undermining and tension on wound closure. Associated sepsis needs antibiotic treatment.

Late/long-term complications

- Wound/breast infection: any collection should be aspirated/drained and appropriate antibiotics commenced. If an implant is *in situ,* it may ultimately need to be removed to eradicate the infection.
- Seroma: a collection of lymphatic/tissue fluid arising in the breast or axilla following removal of the drains. Almost universal after axillary surgery. Does not need draining unless tense and uncomfortable, as aspiration carries a small risk of introducing infection.
- Anaesthesia of the armpit and/or paraesthesia of the inner aspect of the arm after axillary dissection. Due to damage to the second intercostobrachial nerve. Common (up to 80% of women) and not alarming. It may improve gradually for up to 2 years.
- Stiff or frozen shoulder after axillary surgery. This may be prevented by early exercise and physiotherapy.
- Arm lymphoedema occurs in 5–50% of women following axillary surgery as a result of disruption to the afferent lymphatics and the venous drainage of the limb. Active management of this, including referral to specialist lymphoedema services, is important to minimize long-term morbidity. Treatment includes manual lymphatic drainage, massage, arm elevation, and compression garments. It is often noticed following minor trauma to the arm. Therefore, women are advised to avoid having blood taken, injections, or even blood pressure monitored on the operated arm. Patients should protect their affected arm by wearing gloves while doing gardening or activities likely to break the skin.
- Breast lymphoedema is less common but often seen in the medial quadrant of the breast following radiotherapy, infection, haematoma, or large seroma.
- Poor cosmetic result.

Following reconstructive or plastic surgery

- Donor site morbidity after flap surgery. This is often forgotten about; however, tethering following latissimus dorsi and dog ears after TRAM flaps are not uncommon and may need secondary surgery to improve the situation.

Following radiotherapy

With modern machinery, increased fractionation, better planning of radiotherapy, and the use of tangential fields, the incidence of post-radiotherapy complications is decreasing. Some of the rarer complications only present long after the treatment has ended, but the benefits of radiotherapy (decreased local recurrence and a smaller increase in survival) are generally felt to outweigh the risks.

Systemic effects

- Loss of appetite and nausea are uncommon. Fatigue may occur (usually with prior chemotherapy).

Local effects

Short-term

- Skin: reduced basal cell turnover with ongoing epidermal shedding gives rise to epidermal thinning and occasionally progresses to moist desquamation. Erythema occurs when blood vessels become leaky, and some people develop pruritus. These effects settle within 2 weeks (skin turnover time), but hyperpigmentation (from melanocyte stimulation) can last for several months. Good skin care may help.
- Breast: aches and pains within the breast (often mild) can begin with treatment but continue afterwards.
- Shoulder: temporary shoulder restriction is common, possibly due to inflammation or atrophy of the pectoral and rotator cuff muscles. Physiotherapy helps to minimize this effect.
- Oesophagus: occasional oesophagitis with treatment to the central area of the chest.

Long-term

- Skin: damage to endothelial cells and connective tissue gives rise to telangiectasia, and tissues heal poorly with subsequent surgery. Cutaneous radionecrosis is now rare.
- Breast: fibrosis produces a smaller, harder breast that does not alter with time like the contralateral breast. This can give a deteriorating cosmetic result. Irradiation of a reconstructed breast may significantly affect its long-term appearance.
- Arm lymphoedema: occurs following fibrosis and damage to lymphatics and veins. Management of the axilla with radiotherapy alone has a similar risk of arm lymphoedema to that of a standard axillary dissection (5%). Adding radiotherapy to a fully dissected axilla should be avoided, unless there is a high risk of axillary recurrence (e.g. with extensive extracapsular tumour deposition), as the risk of subsequent arm lymphoedema is up to 40%.
- Breast lymphoedema: generally on the medial aspect of the breast and is less common.
- Chest wall: rib pain and occasional rib fracture (<2%) may occur. Osteoradionecrosis is now rare but can arise in patients treated many years ago.

- Lung: radiation pneumonitis, presenting with a dry cough or shortness of breath is rare (0.5%) with breast or chest wall radiotherapy alone but increases if the axilla or supraclavicular fossa (SCF) are also irradiated. It often settles spontaneously.
- Heart: with the use of modern tangential fields, only a small part of the left anterior descending coronary artery is included in the radiotherapy field for left-sided breast cancers, so the risks of cardiac damage are low.
- Brachial plexus: damage to the brachial plexus, causing tingling, numbness, pain, weakness or even paralysis, is uncommon and usually occurs as a result of overlapping fields and high treatment doses.
- Sarcomas: radiation-induced bone or soft tissue sarcomas are rare.

Following systemic therapies

Hormonal manipulation

There are some side effects common to all treatments (although not all women experience all of these effects) and some which are treatment-specific.

Adverse effects common to all treatments

- Hot flushes and sweats.
- Fatigue and mood disturbance.
- Fluid retention, weight gain, and bloating.
- Vaginal discharge, itching, or dryness.
- Irregular periods or amenorrhoea in pre-menopausal women.
- Flare reaction and possible hypercalcaemia with bony metastases.
- Headache, arthralgia, rash, and/or nausea are less common.

Associated with tamoxifen

- Increased risk of endometrial cancer (absolute risk of 0.2%, i.e. a doubling of baseline risk with 5 years of treatment).
- Increased risk of thromboembolic events, deep vein thrombosis (DVT), pulmonary embolism (PE), and cerebrovascular accidents (CVA) (2%).
- Visual disturbance due to cataracts, corneal changes, and rare cases of retinopathy (<1%).
- Thrombocytopenia, leucopenia, liver enzyme changes.
- Contraindicated if pregnant or breastfeeding.

Associated with aromatase inhibitors (AIs)

Although the AIs have a similar adverse effect profile to tamoxifen as outlined, the recent ATAC trial has shown a statistically significant reduction in vaginal discharge, vaginal bleeding, ischaemic cerebrovascular events, and thromboembolic events in patients taking the non-steroidal aromatase inhibitor anastrozole, as opposed to tamoxifen, whilst, conversely, these women appear to be statistically more likely to develop fractures or musculoskeletal disorders (see Further reading for adverse events associated with taximofen and anastrozole.). The size of any long-term clinical difference is awaited.

- All the AIs can cause some gastrointestinal (GI) symptoms (diarrhoea or constipation).
- Anastrozole can lead to increased total cholesterol levels.
- All patients starting an AI need a baseline DEXA scan to assess bone density and the need for adjuvant bone health therapy (see Further Reading).

Associated with oophorectomy (surgical or medical with goserelin)

- Infertility (may be temporary with goserelin).
- Loss of bone mineral density.

Chemotherapy

Neutropenic sepsis is a real and significant danger to patients on chemotherapy. Therefore, it is important they and their GP are aware of the potential symptoms and how to access prompt medical assessment.

Short-term toxicities

Depends on the dose and drug combination used.

- Fatigue and lethargy (80%).
- Nausea and vomiting, eased by anti-emetics.
- Alopecia, reduced risk with use of 'cold cap'.
- Diarrhoea.
- Weight gain (50%) often aggravated by steroids.
- Myelosuppression.
- Infection.
- Mucositis.
- Neuropathy, especially with taxanes.
- Cardiac arrhythmias, cardiac failure with anthracyclines.
- Thromboembolism.
- Allergic reactions with taxanes.

Long-term toxicities

These are less common.

- Premature ovarian failure: the risk increases with age (>60% over age 40), with menopausal symptoms, accelerated loss of bone mineral density, and infertility in up to 40%.
- Myelodysplasia/leukaemia: rare (1%).
- Cardiomyopathy: with high doses of anthracyclines or anthracyclines in combination with trastuzumab.

Signal transduction inhibitors (trastuzumab/Herceptin®)

Transient adverse effects/most common with first treatment

- Flu-like symptoms, fever, chills (40% at first treatment).
- Nausea.
- Diarrhoea.
- Less frequently headache, dizziness, rash, vomiting, or breathlessness.

Serious adverse effects

- Ventricular dysfunction, congestive cardiac failure (5%). Especially when used in combination with anthracyclines or cyclophosphamide. Left ventricular function (LVF) should be evaluated with echo/MUGA prior to and during treatment, and discontinue with any significant drop in LVF.
- Hypersensitivity reactions, including anaphylaxis, infusion reactions, and pulmonary events (especially in metastatic lung disease). Stop drug if significant dyspnoea or hypotension occurs.

Further reading

NICE Guidelines. Available at: http://www.nice.org.uk/nicemedia/pdf/CG80NICEGuideline.pdf.

NMBRA. Available at: http://webarchive.nationalarchives.gov.uk/20120802111034/http://www.ic.nhs.uk/services/national-clinical-audit-support-programme-ncasp/audit-reports/mastectomy-and-breast-reconstruction

For adverse events associated with taximofen and anastrozole, see: Budzar AU (2004). Data from the arimidex, tamoxifen, alone or in combination (ATAC) trial: implications for use of aromatase inhibitors in 2003. *Clin Cancer Res* **10**, 355S–61S.

Chapter 15

Ward management

Enhanced recovery

The Enhanced Recovery Programme (ERP) is a joint Department of Health and NHS Improvement Programme initiative, which aims to improve patient outcomes after surgery by facilitating recovery. The ERP was initially introduced for colorectal surgery and has since been adopted by other surgical specialties, including breast surgery.

The main elements of the ERP are:

- Preoperative preparation.
- Reduced operative stress.
- Structured pain relief.
- Early mobilization.

The target is to reduce length of stay and maximize the use of resources available.

The implementation of an ERP requires good staff communication, as this is a multidisciplinary process involving GPs, pre-assessment clinic nurses, ward staff, theatre staff, anaesthetists, surgeons, dietitians, and physiotherapists. A key period is the preoperative phase, ensuring that patient health is maximized prior to surgery (e.g. stopping smoking, reducing alcohol intake) and that adequate information is given about the operation and recovery period, allowing patients to understand the concept of enhanced recovery.

Pain management is also an important area, which requires optimization following breast surgery, as it delays mobilization and discharge (see Post-operative care). The UK National Mastectomy and Breast Reconstruction Audit demonstrated that, following mastectomy, 6.2% of patients reported severe post-operative pain and that this increased following breast reconstruction. The use of an analgesic ladder, avoidance of opiate-based analgesia, and specific regional anaesthetic techniques, such as paravertebral blocks, should improve patient outcomes. Avoiding the use of drains may also decrease pain and post-operative complications.

Early discharge

It is recommended that >80% of patients undergoing breast surgery should be discharged within 24 hours of their procedure. Increased utilization of day case procedures is generally preferred by patients and is associated with a Best Practice Tariff.

NHS Improvement, in association with the Association of Breast Surgery and British Association of Day Surgery, have produced a day case/one night breast surgical pathway to facilitate this (see Further reading).

The pathway emphasizes the role of the GP in optimizing preoperative health, the importance of comprehensive patient information both during clinic appointments and at pre-assessment, admission on the day of surgery with minimal starvation times, the use of appropriate anaesthesia and analgesia, and the importance of post-operative information and care following discharge.

Discharge planning should be undertaken at the pre-assessment visit to ensure that there are no delays due to predictable social issues.

Preoperative assessment

Preoperative assessment

The aim is to:
- Quantify the severity of the primary disease and any co-morbidity.
- Decide on suitability for day surgical procedures.
- Optimize the patient prior to surgery.
- Obtain informed consent.
- Mark the patient for surgery.

In general, the presence of breast cancer or any other breast pathology does not itself adversely affect the patient's suitability for surgery, although there are certain exceptions:
- Patients who have recently undergone chemotherapy (within 4 weeks) may be neutropenic and at increased risk of post-operative infection. An FBC is essential prior to surgery.
- Prior breast or chest wall radiotherapy increases the chance of post-operative difficulties with wound healing.
- Metastatic breast cancer can cause hypercalcaemia or lung deposits, which may make general anaesthesia risky. Serum calcium level and a CXR should be checked if such metastatic disease is suspected.

Other coexisting medical conditions should be dealt with in the standard fashion. Only age, diabetes, and drugs will be considered further.

Age

Although age itself is not an independent risk factor, it is often accompanied by other health problems, with an increased peri-operative morbidity. Thus, many units have a policy of leaving the axilla untouched in a patient with breast cancer over the age of 80 with no clinical evidence of axillary disease.

Diabetes

Breast surgery is classed as 'minor' surgery for diabetics in that they can eat within 6 hours of the procedure.
- All patients should have BMs monitored at least four times on the day of surgery and hourly if on a sliding scale.
- Assuming adequate control (BMs 4–14), two measurements on the first day post-operatively are usually sufficient.
- Diabetics should be first on the operating list where possible.
- Patients on diet treatment (or metformin) only should fast as required for surgery and avoid 5% glucose as fluid replacement intra-operatively.
- Patients on other oral hypoglycaemic drugs should omit these tablets on the morning of surgery. After recovery, they can have a light meal and their normal oral hypoglycaemics.
- Insulin-dependent diabetics: omit morning insulin. Start insulin sliding scale at least 2 hours prior to theatre. Restart normal insulin regimen once eating and drinking.

Drugs

Tamoxifen is usually withheld prior to surgery to decrease the risk of venous thromboembolism. Warfarin, clopidogrel, and aspirin should be stopped prior to surgery. In high-risk patients (e.g. metallic heart valves or recent coronary stenting), anticoagulation should be discussed with the cardiology team and a treatment plan documented prior to surgery. Most hospitals have an anticoagulant pathway for patients on long-term anti-coagulation, whereby the anticoagulation team formulates a plan for the patient covering the whole peri-operative period.

Preoperative investigations

- In benign disease in a young patient with no significant medical history, 'routine' tests are not needed. Unfortunately, these patients are rare.
- Afro-Caribbeans should be tested for sickle cell trait.
- Mediterraneans need to have thalassaemia excluded.
- FBC prior to all breast cancer procedures and G&S prior to mastectomy/axillary clearance and all reconstructive procedures.
- Clotting studies in those on anticoagulants or with known liver impairment.
- U&E on diabetics, patients with renal impairment, or those on drugs causing electrolyte disturbance (e.g. diuretics, digoxin, steroids).
- CXR in those with a history suggestive of symptomatic cardiorespiratory disease or possible lung metastases. Not required in women <60 years with early-stage breast cancer.
- ECG in patients >50 years, diabetics >40 years, or patients with any cardiac history.

Preoperative preparations for theatre

Thromboprophylaxis

There is an increased risk of DVT and PE in women with malignancy, especially those having long reconstructive operations. The risk is increased in women on tamoxifen or those who have recently had chemotherapy. Thus, all women with no contraindications should receive TED stockings, with or without a low molecular weight heparin. Pneumatic compression devices are routinely used in theatres, and the patients are encouraged to be up and mobile as soon as possible after surgery.

Consent

The surgeon performing the operation, or an assistant who is familiar with the procedure, should take consent. This issue has been extensively covered elsewhere, so suffice it to say that decisions about the exact nature of the breast, axillary, and reconstructive surgery to be undertaken are often complex and should have been thoroughly discussed with the patient prior to admission.

Marking the patient

This should be done by the surgeon on the ward.

- The side of the surgery (and indicate what operation is to be performed).
- The site of incisions (drawn with patient standing in order to get scars in a skin crease or inframammary crease).
- The borders of the breast (to prevent removal of excess tissue and facilitate re-shaping).
- Skin excisions and flaps.
- Midline and contralateral breast (to allow symmetrization).

Antibiotic prophylaxis

The majority of patients undergoing breast surgery will benefit from peri-operative prophylactic antibiotics. Local antibiotic policy based upon local microbiological preferences and sensitivities should be adhered to. Prophylaxis should be given against MRSA for those previously exposed or currently colonized. Prolonged prophylaxis should be considered in patients undergoing implant surgery.

Always go and see the patient yourself before the patient has been anaesthetized. You should check the following:

- Is the lesion palpable with the patient lying as they would be on the operating table? If not, should it be localized?
- Has the lesion grown? If yes, is the planned surgery, i.e. breast-conserving, still possible?
- Does the patient understand what procedure they are about to undergo?
- Does the patient agree with the site of the lesion?

- Consent and mark the patient. In some instances, this is best done with the patient supine, in others (e.g. mastopexy) with the patient sitting.
- Check that FNA, core biopsy, and routine blood results are in the notes. Ensure mammograms are available. Blood has been grouped or cross-matched, if necessary.
- Antibiotics, TED stockings, and heparin prophylaxis should be prescribed as required by local policy.

Post-operative care

General measures

- Patients can generally eat, drink, and mobilize soon after surgery.
- Wounds can be washed in the shower from the first post-operative day but should be dried gently and not left covered in damp dressings; a hairdryer may be helpful.
- Pressure dressings should be removed in order to inspect the wound on the first post-operative day. After this, clean, dry wounds can be left open or a simple Mepore® dressing applied.
- A soft bra can be worn when comfortable.
- Drains are generally left *in situ* until draining less than 30–50mL of serosanguinous fluid/day or at day 5 (whichever comes first). However, many units are happy for patients to go home with their drains, and the community nurses will monitor the drainage and remove when ready.
- Physiotherapy should be initiated prior to discharge to encourage a range of exercises to keep the arm and shoulder moving.
- Advice on arm and skin care after axillary surgery.
- Ensure patients have contact numbers for breast care nurse in case of physical/emotional problems.
- Post-operative haemoglobin may be necessary, following mastectomies, reconstructions, or major cosmetic procedures.
- Check wound for haematoma, flaps/nipples for evidence of necrosis.
- The breast care nurse should see the patient regarding the fitting of a prosthesis.
- Arrange first post-operative follow-up.

Pain management

Pain control after breast surgery was assessed in the National Mastectomy and Breast Reconstruction Audit (see Further reading). Significant levels of post-operative pain were experienced, and conclusions of the audit were that units should be auditing pain control and improving peri-operative analgesia. Methods of pain control peri-operatively include:

Analgesia

- Paracetamol.
- Non-steroidal anti-inflammatory drugs.
- Oral opiates, e.g. codeine (these should always be given in conjunction with aperients and anti-emetics).
- IV opiates, such as pethidine (short-acting) and morphine (long-acting), with an anti-emetic.

Local anaesthetic

- Peri-operative injection to wound surfaces, including all raw surfaces.
- Peri-operative infiltration down a drain.
- Wound infiltration catheters.
- Blockade: paravertebral, intercostal, and interpleural blocks are used for breast surgery.

Flap management

Patients having complex reconstructive procedures need careful observation of the flap for the first few hours/days.

- Ensure good oxygenation.
- Good analgesia to avoid hypertension.
- Keep the patient warm, gamgee on the flap, a warming blanket on the patient.
- Obtain IV access, and keep well perfused with good urine output (50mL/h)—catheters are useful following flap surgery.
- Avoid smoking.
- Abdominal wall flaps (TRAM/DIEP) require a period of bed rest, with hip and knee flexion before mobilization.

Physiotherapy

Begins on day 1 post-operatively, with a respiratory assessment and the teaching of breathing exercises to minimize the effects of anaesthesia and shoulder exercises to restore movement and function to the arm as soon as possible. After a full axillary clearance, physiotherapy can also reduce the risk of lymphoedema. The exercises are repeated two to three times daily for at least 6 weeks or until a full range of movement is regained. (Additional physiotherapy during radiotherapy may minimize shoulder stiffness). They include:

- Shoulder circling.
- Hair brushing.
- Back scratching.
- Arm bending.
- Arm lifts.
- Wall climbing.
- Back drying.

Cancer pain and its management

In general, breast cancer is not painful, unless it invades a nerve or due to bulk compressing and pressure effects.

- Oral analgesics are the mainstay of pain relief in patients with cancer. Strong opioids are safe and effective for moderate to severe pain.
- Analgesia should be taken regularly at prescribed times, rather than on an as-needed (PRN) basis. PRN analgesics for chronic pain should be reserved for breakthrough pain only.
- Radiotherapy plays a major role in the management of acute cancer pain.
- The regular use of laxatives should be considered in conjunction with the administration of analgesics, preferably before constipation develops.
- Bisphosphonates have a role in the treatment and prevention of bone pain in breast cancer.
- Non-steroidal anti-inflammatory drugs have a role in the treatment of inflammatory or bone pain.
- Epidural, intrathecal, and intracerebroventricular opioids are often effective in treating acute pain that is not controlled with conventional treatment.

Further reading

NHS Institute for Innovation and Improvement: Quality and Service Improvement Tool. Available at: http://www.institute.nhs.uk/quality_and_service_improvement_tools/quality_and_service_improvement_tools/enhanced_recovery_programme.html

NHS Enhanced Recovery Partnership. Available at: http://www.improvement.nhs.uk/enhancedrecovery2/Breast.aspx.

National Mastectomy and Breast Reconstruction Audit 2010. Available at: http://www.ic.nhs.uk/services/national-clinical-audit-support-programme-ncasp/audit-reports/mastectomy-and-breast-reconstruction

Arsalani-Zadeh R, ElFadl D, Yassin N, MacFie J (2011). Evidence-based review of enhancing postoperative recovery after breast surgery. *Br J Surg* **98**, 181–96.

Breast Cancer Care. Available at: http://www.breastcancercare.org.uk

NMBRA. Available at: http://webarchive.nationalarchives.gov.uk/20120802111034/http://www.ic.nhs.uk/services/national-clinical-audit-support-programme-ncasp/audit-reports/mastectomy-and-breast-reconstruction

NHS Improvement in association with the Association of Breast Surgery and British Association of Day Surgery, a day case/one night breast surgical pathway (Dec 2011). Available at: http://www.improvement.nhs.uk/documents/DayCaseBreastSurgery.pdf

Chapter 16

Breast reduction

Breast reduction

Basic principles

Breast reduction surgery is cosmetic surgery performed to decrease the size of a breast. The majority of cases are performed bilaterally to reduce the size of the breasts when their size causes significant symptoms for the patient. Breast reduction surgery involves moving breast parenchyma and nipples on pedicles carrying their blood supply. The principles of this surgery will prepare a breast trainee for volume displacement techniques in breast conservation and therapeutic mammaplasty (see Chapter 18). Breast reduction is the basis of much of oncoplastic breast surgery. Breast reduction surgery improves quality of life to a similar extent to that observed in hip replacement surgery (see Further reading).

Common reasons for seeking breast reduction surgery include:

- Associated back/neck/shoulder pain caused by the breast weight.
- Unwanted attention due to the size of the cleavage.
- Difficulty with hygiene due to breast size/ptosis.
- Psychological impact of having large breasts.
- To aid symmetry following previous contralateral mastectomy/breast reconstruction surgery.
- Massive breast hypertrophy during pregnancy.

The aims of breast reduction surgery include four core principles (see Further reading):

- Excision of excess parenchyma: excess parenchyma must be removed whilst leaving adequate breast tissue to maintain a suitable final breast size for the patient's body shape and to maintain bulk in the medial cleavage region.
- Skin envelope reduction: when reducing breast bulk, it is usually necessary to remove skin excess to reduce breast ptosis and to help maintain breast shape long-term.
- Breast shaping: the final result must give good long-term breast shape, with nipples placed at an appropriate height upon a well-projected breast mound.
- Nipple complex blood and nerve supply: the nipple vascularity and sensation are preserved by fashioning a pedicle of breast tissue large enough to support nipple viability.

From the patient's point of view, breast reduction surgery carries the advantages of:

- Reduced breast bulk.
- Improved breast ptosis and shape.

Against this has to be weighed the disadvantages of:

- Scarring to the breast.
- Changes caused to breast appearance on mammography.
- Future ability to breastfeed may be prevented.
- Reduced nipple sensation/erotic sensation.

All breast reconstruction surgery is potentially prone to complications, but particular caution has to be exercised in the face of:

- Previous radiotherapy.
- Smokers/vascular disease/diabetics.
- Previous breast augmentation/breast reduction.

Preoperative discussion and assessment

Before accepting a patient for breast reduction, it is important to get a clear picture of the patient's motivations behind seeking surgery and their expectations of the final result. Breast reduction surgery carries significant risk of complications, which the patient must be made fully aware of. It should not be seen as a simple cosmetic procedure. The most serious potential complication is nipple and fat necrosis, which can result in complete loss of the central breast tissue and significant breast deformity.

Therefore, the preoperative assessment of the patient needs to include both the previous medical and social history. In particular, disorders associated with problems in tissue perfusion and increased risk of infection, together with smoking, heavy alcohol, or other social drug use, are relative contraindications to surgery because of the potential disturbance to vascularity.

Physical assessment of the patient needs to include measurements of the suprasternal to nipple distance and the nipple to inframammary fold since it is these measurements that will be used in preoperative marking. The breast needs assessing for any evidence of pathology and, in ladies over 40, a mammogram should be obtained. Preoperative photographs must be obtained.

Complications and consent issues

Patients must be made aware of the risks and complications, both at the preoperative discussion and at the time consent is obtained. It is often helpful to reiterate these in correspondence with the GP and the patient. Reduction surgery is a happy hunting ground for medical negligence lawyers and their expert witness henchmen, and they will seize on any slight chink in the informed consent process to ensure a successful payout.

The important points to emphasize and include in the consent process are:

- The surgeon is unable to guarantee a cup size of the breast that will be achieved post-operatively.
- Visible scars on the breast, which can become hypertrophic/keloid.
- Infection.
- Bleeding and possible return to theatre.
- Wound dehiscence (most commonly at the junction of the 'T').
- Fat necrosis (development of lumps requiring triple assessment or, if the fat necrosis is superficial, it presents with oily discharge).
- Asymmetry.
- Numbness or occasionally hyperaesthesia of the nipple-areola complex.
- Chronic pain.
- Partial, or total, loss of the nipple complex because of necrosis.

- Incomplete relief of symptoms, such as back pain.
- Breast reduction causes mammographic changes to the breast, which may require further assessment following breast screening.
- Interference with ability to breastfeed in the future.
- Relapse with the breast increasing in size again, particularly with weight gain.

Photographs should be taken before and after surgery, and any preoperative asymmetry should be pointed out to the patient.

Patients should be shown photographs, with a range of outcomes experienced following breast reduction surgery.

Operative techniques

Patients must be aware of all the options available, including having no surgery or attempting weight loss to reduce breast bulk.

The techniques available should be discussed with the patient, including Wise pattern (inverted T), vertical pattern, peri-areolar scarring, and breast liposuction.

Several techniques exist, of which the commonest in use is probably the Wise pattern approach. It is important to match the most appropriate procedure to the patient, not the patient to the procedure that you are familiar with.

- Wise pattern: the most commonly used skin pattern with predictable results and immediately good breast shape in most patients. The Wise pattern deals well with skin excess and ptosis. It can be used with any pedicle.
- Vertical pattern: this results in a peri-areolar scar with a lower vertical extension. Vertical scar reductions eliminate the horizontal scar of the inverted T techniques. Approximately 10–20% of patients will require scar revision to eliminate a dog ear at the inferior end of the scar. Revision often requires a short horizontal scar. These are best used for smaller reductions on young women with good quality skin. Long-term results are excellent, but the optimal shape is not achieved for approximately 3 months. Lejour, Hall–Findlay, and Lassus techniques are variations of the vertical reduction, which utilize superior or superomedial pedicles.
- Peri-areolar: the round block reduction (Benelli) limits scars to a peri-areolar scar. It can be used selectively for young patients and is best performed in those requiring small reductions. A superior pedicle is most commonly used, and a non-absorbable suture is used subcutaneously to try to stop the areola from enlarging over time. Initially, the peri-areolar skin will be ruffled, but this usually settles over the following months. Patients must be aware that a proportion of patients will need revisional surgery with conversion to a vertical/Wise pattern technique.

- Breast liposuction: removes bulk from the breast but does not address ptosis or skin redundancy. It is of limited use in older women who have predominantly fatty breasts. Liposuction has the advantage of removing mass without significant scars. The most common complication of breast liposuction is haematoma formation (1–3%).
- Free nipple graft: it is useful for patients with enormous breasts that would end up with a pedicle that is too long. It is a good technique in older women who may have a diminished microvasculature. It is easy to perform and gives additional flexibility in shaping the breast because the pedicle does not need preserving as in most other techniques. The major drawback is that the nipple appearance may be poor and is without sensation.

Marking of a patient for Wise pattern breast reduction

There are many different ways to mark patients for breast reduction. The Wise pattern is easily followed, can be replicated, and gives consistently good aesthetic results (see Fig. 16.1). It is vital that the surgeon performing the operation marks the patient. The patient must be standing or sitting on the side of the bed; trying to mark the patient on their back or asleep in theatre will result in complete disaster. The indefensible complication is if the final position of the nipple is too high and coming out of the bra, so it is recommended to follow these steps:

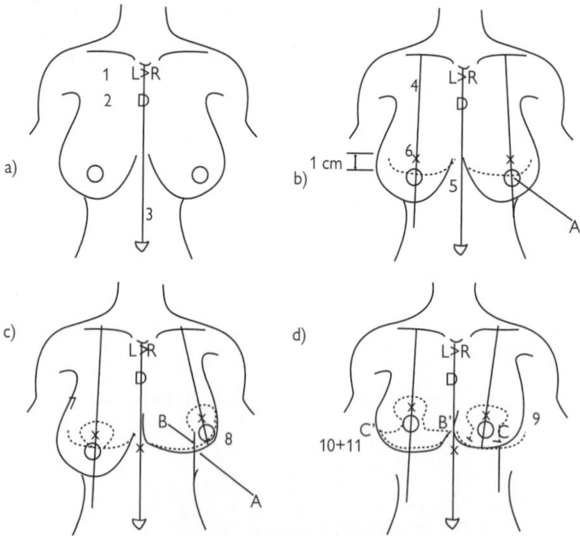

Fig. 16.1 Marking of a Wise pattern breast reduction. a) 1. Any preoperative breast asymmetry is marked on the patient. 2. Desired final cup size (not guaranteed, just a guide) is marked. 3. Midline is marked, including suprasternal notch. b) 4. With a tape measure around the neck, the breast meridian is drawn. 5. Level of the inframammary fold (IMF) is marked on the midline. 6. One cm above the IMF, the new nipple site is marked on the line of the breast meridian. c) 7. Outline of new areola is marked. 8. Lift the breast, and push laterally; mark a plumb line between the medial edge of the marked areola (B) and the midpoint of the inframammary fold (A). d) 9. Lift the breast, and push medially; mark a plumb line between the lateral edge of the marked areola (C) and the midpoint of the inframammary fold (A). 10, 11. Place a thumb midway between points A + B (and A + C); fold the breast until these two points are touching. Where the crease of skin folding meets the inframammary fold is the medial and lateral (respectively) extents of the Wise pattern incisions. Mark the inframammary fold, and join B to B' and C to C'.

1. With the patient standing, assess the patient's breast size. If one breast is larger and needs more reduction, write this on the patient's sternum.
2. Write the patient's aim for final cup size over sternum.
3. Mark suprasternal notch and midline along sternum and down to umbilicus.
4. Put a tape measure around the patient's neck, so it falls over the current nipple site. Draw breast meridian along the tape measure through the current nipple and down the breast to cross the inframammary fold.
5. Place a finger in the inframammary fold, and translate this level across to the midline and make a mark on the midline. Put fingers in the inframammary fold and thumb on the anterior surface of breast (Pitanguy's point), and mark this point on the midline. This should correspond with your first mark.
6. The centre of the new nipple site should be 1–3cm above this height. One cm above this mark, draw the new nipple height on the breast meridian bilaterally. Measure from the suprasternal notch to the new nipple height. This distance should NEVER be less than 21cm and only less than 23cm in a very small-framed woman. Ensure bilateral measurements are the same.
7. Draw the new areola margin around the new nipple site. If your nipple marker is 4cm in diameter, this areola margin needs to be $2 \times \pi \times$ radius = 12.5cm in length. Check the length of this ellipse with a tape measure. Alternatively, use a template to draw this elliptical shape.
8. Place a thumb just medial to the nipple, and move the breast gently upwards and laterally so that the redundant skin is taken up and the ptosis is removed. Draw a line vertically down from the medial areolar edge towards the intercept of the breast meridian with the inframammary fold (point A). Put a mark 5.5cm down this line (point B).
9. Place a thumb just lateral to the nipple, and move the breast gently upwards and medially so that the redundant skin is taken up and the ptosis is removed. Draw a line vertically down from the lateral areolar edge towards the intercept of the breast meridian with the inframammary fold (point A). Put a mark at 5.5cm down this line (point C).
10. Place a thumb halfway between point B and the inframammary fold. Using your fingers, fold the breast over so that point B comes and rests over point A. There will now be a crease in the skin that extends to the medial aspect of the inframammary fold. Mark this most medial point of the skin incision (B'). Let go of the breast, and draw a straight line from point B to B'.
11. Place a thumb halfway between point C and point A. Using your fingers, fold the breast over so that point C comes and rests over point A. There will now be a crease in the skin that extends to the lateral aspect of the inframammary fold. Mark this point (C'). Let go of the breast, and draw a straight line from point C to C'. Mark the inframammary fold from point B' to C'. Points B' and C' should not meet in the middle and should be at least 3cm apart to avoid synmastia.
12. Stand back, and ensure markings are symmetrical.

Post-operative care

Patients will usually have a drain placed post-reduction surgery. This drain does not avoid bleeding problems, but does allow earlier detection of a bleed, and avoids the pedicle being compressed by an expanding haematoma before the patient is returned to the operating theatre. The drain can be safely removed the day following surgery. Patients are advised to wear a soft sports bra, day and night for the first 4 weeks after surgery, and to moisturize their scars on a daily basis once healed.

The commonest immediate complication is a haematoma, which invariably needs evacuating. It is important to treat signs of infection early, as failure to do so can encourage fat necrosis in the pedicle which then causes nipple necrosis.

Further reading

Jones GE, ed (2010). *Bostwick's plastic and reconstructive breast surgery*, 3e. Quality Medical Publishing, St Louis.

Spear SL, Willey SC, Robb GL, Hammond DC, Nahabedian MY, eds (2010). *Surgery of the breast: principles and art*, 3e. Lippincott Williams & Wilkins, Philadelphia.

Chapter 17

Oncoplastic mastectomy incisions

Overview

The best cosmesis following mastectomy is achieved by maintaining the original skin envelope of the breast, including the nipple. Not all patients are oncologically suitable for a skin-sparing or nipple-sparing mastectomy. Preoperative planning is essential for all patients having a mastectomy so that the optimum aesthetic outcome can be achieved in either an immediate or a delayed reconstructive setting.

Simple mastectomy incisions

Simple mastectomy incisions should be designed to maximize the cosmetic outcome should a patient choose to have a reconstruction in the delayed setting. In designing the incision, we should attempt to:

- Keep the scar as low on the breast as possible, so it is not visible.
- Ensure that skin in the décolleté/cleavage region is intact and the medial end of the scar is low.
- If possible, maintain the inframammary fold and its attachments. In a ptotic breast, the upper flap can be sutured at the level of the inframammary fold (see Fig. 17.1). This ensures that, in a delayed reconstruction, the skin paddle from an autologous reconstruction is hidden in the inferior pole of the breast, and the visible part of the breast is native skin.

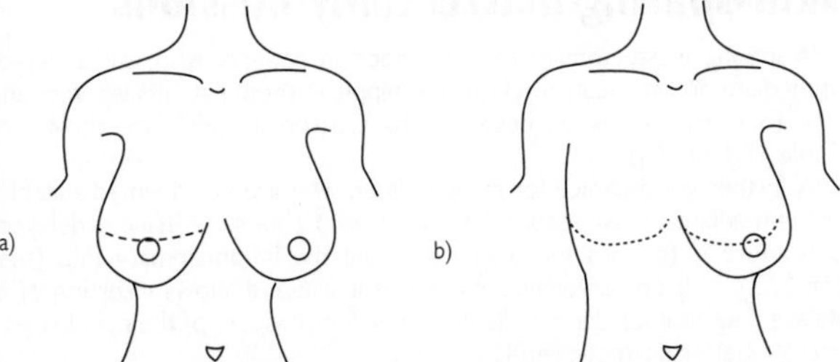

Fig. 17.1 Maintaining the inframammary fold during simple mastectomy. a) In the ptotic breast, the upper flap is marked as low as possible, just above the nipple (incisions marked with a dashed line). The lower skin incision is made at the level of the inframammary fold, care being taken to maintain the attachments of the fascial layers at this level. b) The upper flap is brought down following the mastectomy and sutured at the level of the inframammary fold.

Skin-sparing mastectomy incisions

Skin-sparing mastectomies are performed in patients who will undergo immediate breast reconstruction. The nipple in these patients is removed. The four main types, as described by Carlson in 1997, are shown in Table 17.1 and Fig. 17.2.

A further good choice for many women who are not deemed suitable for immediate breast reconstruction or who choose to have a delayed procedure is to conserve breast skin and the inframammary fold (see Fig. 17.2). This preserves upper chest wall skin and allows insertion of a delayed autologous skin paddle into the inferior aspect of the new breast, giving a better cosmetic result.

Table 17.1 Common incision types used for skin-sparing mastectomies

Type	Incision
I	Peri-areolar incision (with or without a lateral extension)—this incision can be closed with a purse string suture, or a paddle from an autologous flap can be inset into this space.
II	A peri-areolar incision, incorporating skin over superficial tumours or an adjacent biopsy/wide local excision scar on the breast.
III	A peri-areolar incision—the skin overlying superficial tumours or previous surgery sites is removed without excising the intervening skin.
IV	The nipple-areola complex is removed, using an inverted T or Wise pattern reduction scar.

This classification includes incisions required in patients following a previous attempt at breast-conserving surgery.

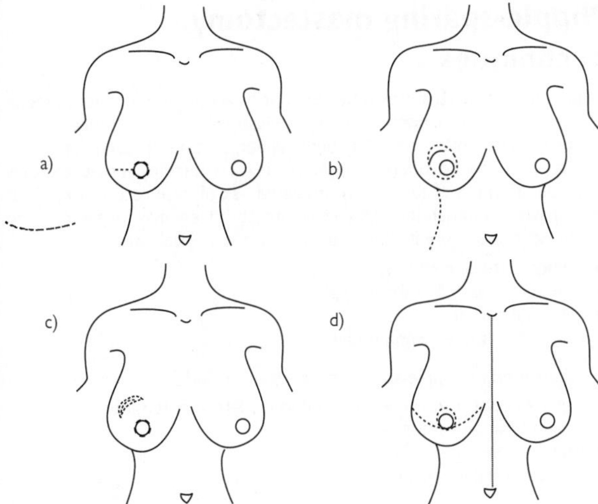

Fig. 17.2 Skin-sparing mastectomy incisions. a) Type I incision—peri-areolar, with or without a lateral extension. b) Type II incision—to include the nipple and a previous lumpectomy scar. c) Type III incisions—both the nipple and lumpectomy scars are excised separately. d) Type IV Wise pattern incision.

Nipple-sparing mastectomy techniques

Nipple-sparing mastectomy is becoming increasingly common for immediate breast reconstructions and is an excellent choice for women undergoing prophylactic mastectomy. Patients undergoing mastectomy for breast cancer can also be offered nipple-sparing mastectomy; however, they must be informed of the slightly increased risk of local recurrence. Spear *et al.* have recommended that certain breast cancers may be amenable to nipple-sparing surgery if they meet specific oncological criteria:

- Tumour size 3cm or less.
- Tumour at least 2cm from nipple.
- Not multicentric.
- Clinically negative lymph nodes.

Incisions used for nipple-sparing mastectomy include:

- A peri-areolar incision (with or without a lateral extension).
- A lateral radial incision.
- An inframammary incision.
- A reduction pattern incision.

The safety of nipple-sparing mastectomy may be increased by obtaining nipple shaves at the time of surgery or by taking core biopsies from behind the nipple prior to the mastectomy.

Specific risks of skin-sparing or nipple-sparing mastectomy

- Flap necrosis: the longer flaps used in this surgery will cause an increased risk of skin flap necrosis. This risk is highest if using reduction pattern surgery. Careful planning of skin incision type is essential in all patients, particularly those already at higher risk of necrosis (prior radiotherapy, smokers, vascular disease, diabetics). Leaving skin bridges (type III skin-sparing mastectomy) may not be advisable in this cohort of high-risk patients.
- Higher risk of locally recurrent disease: the more skin and nipple that is spared, potentially the more breast tissue will be left behind. This will put patients at higher risk of locally recurrent disease or, in the the prophylactic setting, of developing a primary breast cancer.
- Partial or total nipple necrosis if the nipple is being spared.
- Loss of sensation: this occurs to the breast skin envelope and also to the nipple if spared.

Further reading

Rainsbury D, Willett A (2012). Oncoplastic breast reconstruction—Guidelines for Best Practice ABS/BAPRAS Nov 2012. Available at: http://www.associationofbreastsurgery.org.uk/media/23851/final_oncoplastic_guidelines_for_use.pdf

Spear SL, Willey SC, Robb GL, Hammond DC, Nahabedian MY, eds (2010). *Surgery of the breast: principles and art*, 3e. Lippincott Williams & Wilkins, Philadelphia.

Carlson GW, Bostwick J 3rd, Styblo TM, *et al.* (1997). Skin-sparing mastectomy. Oncologic and reconstructive consideration. *Ann Surg* **225**, 570–5.

Hannan C, Spear S, Seiboth L, Al-Attar A (2010). Nipple sparing mastectomy: A review on indications, techniques and safety. *Plast Reconstr Surg* **126**, 25.

National Mastectomy and Breast Reconstruction Audits. Available at: http://www.ic.nhs.uk/services/national-clinical-audit-support-programme-ncasp/audit-reports/mastectomy-and-breast-reconstruction

Jones GE, ed (2010). *Bostwick's plastic and reconstructive breast surgery*, 3e. Quality Medical Publishing, St Louis.

Chapter 18

Breast-conserving surgery: volume displacement

Overview

Breast-conserving surgery (BCS), combined with radiotherapy, has equivalent survival rates to mastectomy. The goal is to conserve breast shape whilst removing an adequate volume of tissue.

When >20% of breast volume is excised during wide local excision, there is a higher risk of developing deformity of the breast. This can be distressing for the patient and may require multiple operations in an attempt to restore normal breast form.

Classification of post-WLE deformities

Deformities can be classified for descriptive purposes, although how they are managed must be based on individual assessment.

- Grade 1: loss of volume—requires local flap or lipomodelling.
- Grade 2: loss of volume and ptosis—requires contralateral symmetrization.
- Grade 3: loss of shape—requires scar revision or local remodelling.
- Grade 4: loss of shape and volume—requires volume replacement.
- Grade 5: extensive fibrosis—requires mastectomy and reconstruction.

Oncoplastic breast-conserving surgery (OBCS)

The initial use of oncoplastic breast-conserving techniques will minimize the risk of post-operative breast deformities and should be considered for all resections >20% of breast volume. Tumours in the lower and medial poles of the breast are particularly prone to post-operative deformity.

The principles of OBCS are the same as for standard WLE—to excise at least a margin of normal tissue around the tumour, taking a full thickness of tissue from the level of skin down to pectoralis fascia. The cavity should be clipped to facilitate radiotherapy prior to remodelling.

Patient factors are important in deciding on the appropriate technique. All patients should be counselled about the risks of poor scarring and post-operative breast asymmetry. Contralateral symmetrization may be required, either immediately or as a second-stage procedure following completion of adjuvant treatment.

Techniques fall into two broad groups:

- Volume displacement—local breast tissue is mobilized to fill the defect and may form part of a breast reduction procedure.
- Volume replacement (see Chapter 19)—new tissue is brought in, often in the form of a myocutaneous flap.

Smoking, diabetes, and high BMI increase the risk of complications, especially wound infections and delayed healing. These patients should be counselled appropriately prior to surgery.

Advantages of OBCS

- No difference in oncological outcome compared to standard WLE.
- Allows larger volume of tissue to be excised.
- Improved cosmetic result.

Disadvantages of OBCS

- Re-excision may be difficult, as original margins not easily identified.
- Increased risk of complications, e.g. fat necrosis.
- Delayed healing will delay adjuvant therapy.

Classification of OBCS

Level 1 techniques:
- Local glandular remodelling.
- Up to 20% volume excision.
- Dual-plane undermining required—glandular breasts only.

Level 2 techniques:
- Mammaplasty techniques.
- 20–50% volume excision, with or without skin excision.
- Single-plane undermining—suitable for fatty and glandular breasts.

Level 1 OBCS techniques

- Mark patient preoperatively in standing position.
- Position patient on operating table to allow an upright position during surgery.
- Drape patient with both breasts exposed.
- Make sufficient skin incision to allow extensive glandular mobilization.
- Undermine skin in mastectomy plane beyond tumour site.
- If necessary, transect nipple ducts, leaving 1cm tissue on underside of NAC to facilitate repositioning.
- Excise full-thickness fusiform wedge of breast tissue, including tumour orientated along breast ray.
- Orientate specimen for pathologist.
- Mark cavity with metal clips.
- Mobilize surrounding breast tissue from pectoralis fascia to create local glandular flaps, and approximate to fill defect.
- If necessary, de-epithelialize crescent of peri-areolar skin opposite excision to re-centre NAC.

Level 2 OBCS techniques

Choice of technique depends on tumour location, but all are variations on basic mammaplasty procedures and allow extensive volume excision along with overlying skin. Appropriate options are summarized in Table 18.1.

The use of level 2 techniques requires specialist training and is based on breast reduction procedures. Details of each procedure will not be covered here but can be found in any good oncoplastic textbook.

- Mark patient preoperatively in standing position.
- Position patient on operating table to allow upright position during surgery.
- Drape patient, with both breasts exposed.
- Incise skin pattern to dermis.
- De-epithelialize nipple pedicle if necessary.
- Perform full-thickness wedge excision of breast tissue, including tumour with overlying skin.
- Mobilize surrounding breast tissue from pectoralis fascia.
- Approximate glandular flaps, and inset nipple pedicle.
- Use of drain is optional.
- Perform contralateral symmetrization if required.

Table 18.1 Level 2 techniques for OBCS

Position of tumour	Suggested procedure
Lower pole	Superior pedicle mammaplasty/Vertical mammaplasty
Upper pole	Inferior pedicle mammaplasty/Round block technique
Medial pole	Medial mammaplasty
Lateral pole	Lateral mammaplasty
Central	Wise pattern mammaplasty including NAC, Vertical mammaplasty including NAC

Further reading

Rainsbury D, Willett A (2012). Oncoplastic breast reconstruction—Guidelines for Best Practice ABS/BAPRAS Nov 2012. Available at: http://www.associationofbreastsurgery.org.uk/media/23851/final_oncoplastic_guidelines_for_use.pdf

Clough KB, Kaufman GJ, Nos C, Buccimazza I, Sarfati IM (2010). Improving breast cancer surgery: a classification and quadrant per quadrant atlas for oncoplastic surgery. *Ann Surg Oncol* **17**, 1375–91.

Fitoussi A, Berry MG, Couturaud B, Salmon RJ (2009). *Oncoplastic and reconstructive surgery for breast cancer.* Springer, London.

Spear SL, Willey SC, Robb GL, Hammond DC, Nahabedian MY, eds (2010). *Surgery of the breast: principles and art*, 3e. Lippincott Williams & Wilkins, Philadelphia.

Iwuchukwu OC, Harvey JR, Dordea M, *et al.* The role of therapeutic mammaplasty in breast cancer surgery—a review. *Surg Oncol* **21**, 133–41.

Jones GE, ed (2010). *Bostwick's plastic and reconstructive breast surgery*, 3e. Quality Medical Publishing, St Louis.

Baildam A (2002). Oncoplastic surgery of the breast. *Br J Surg* **89**, 532–3.

Chapter 19

Breast reconstruction: volume replacement

Overview

Volume replacement should be considered in the setting of:

- Immediate or delayed breast reconstruction after mastectomy.
- >20% of breast volume resected as part of breast-conserving surgery.
- Resection of central, medial, or lower pole tumours likely to cause significant deformity.

Common types of volume replacement

- Implant-based reconstruction.
- Autologous flap reconstruction (e.g. latissimus dorsi, abdominal, or gluteal flap).
- Lipomodelling.

Selection of volume replacement technique

The key to successful volume replacement and patient satisfaction is the clinical decision-making process. Clinician, patient, family, and breast care nurses should be involved in the decision-making process. Patients must be aware:

- Reconstructive surgery is a choice, unlike their cancer surgery.
- It involves risk of complications and prolonged recovery.
- That the complications of reconstructive surgery may delay adjuvant therapies.
- Of all the options available for reconstruction (even if they are not available in your hospital).
- What is involved in each reconstructive option to aid informed decision-making.
- That reconstructive surgery usually involves several operations and multiple clinic visits.
- A reconstructed breast will not be the same as their natural breast.

This process will take multiple visits to achieve understanding and agreement. Specialist nurses are the backbone of this discussion and should be giving patients written information, photographs of a range of reconstructions with a range of outcomes (from good through to those having peri-operative complications), and, if time permits, a meeting with patients who have undergone breast reconstruction.

History-taking

A full medical history should be taken from all patients. Important information includes:

- Previous adjuvant treatment (especially radiotherapy and its dosage).
- Smoking history.
- Current weight and BMI, and stability of current weight (large variations in weight will rapidly change the appearance of the reconstructed vs the non-reconstructed breast).
- Which breast does the patient prefer?
- What does patient want to achieve from breast reconstruction?
- Social history of current job and hobbies (especially sport).
- Family circumstances (e.g. is the patient a carer for young children?).

Clinical examination

Clinical examination should incorporate:

- Recording of BMI.
- Assessment breast shape, including height/width/projection and ptosis.
- Examination of the presence/absence of pectoralis major and latissimus dorsi.
- Assessment of breast/chest wall skin quality and any radiation changes.
- Examination of the abdominal pannus for amount and quality of tissue.
- Examination for abdominal wall hernias or weakness.

Implant-based reconstruction and acellular dermal matrices

Basic principles

A permanent implant or expander is placed in a subpectoral pocket, which covers the superior and medial aspects of the implant. The more tissue covering an implant, the more natural it will feel.

The inferior and lateral aspects of the implant are more difficult to cover. The main options to cover this area include:

- Skin-only coverage (implant may, therefore, be palpable/visible).
- Creating a total submuscular pocket by also lifting serratus anterior.
- Inserting an acellular dermal matrix (e.g. Strattice™) or mesh.
- Using a dermal flap as part of a skin-reducing (e.g. Wise pattern) mastectomy.
- Lifting an abdominal fascial flap, including rectus abdominis and external oblique fascia.

Advantages

- Short operation and recovery. Full recovery takes weeks, not months.
- Gives good results, particularly in small, non-ptotic breasts.
- The use of expander implants gives adjustability.
- Good for patients unwilling to undergo autologous flap reconstruction.

Disadvantages

- Post-operative adjuvant radiotherapy often results in poor cosmesis.
- Risk of implant infection.
- Further revisional operations are usually required.
- Multiple clinic visits are needed for expansion.
- Lack of ptosis—patient may be asymmetrical compared with the contralateral side.
- Cost of acellular dermal matrices.
- Does not provide extra skin often needed in the delayed setting.
- Is not suitable for partial breast reconstruction.
- Long-term development of capsular contracture.

Contraindications

- Sepsis.
- If post-operative radiotherapy is likely (a relative contraindication).
- Thin, damaged, or irradiated skin (a relative contraindication).

Consent

The consent discussion should include discussion about the potential adverse outcomes of implant-based reconstruction, including;

- Likely need for revisional surgery in the future.
- Capsular contracture (the risk increases with time).
- Implant infection and subsequent risk of implant removal.
- Implant extrusion (particular risk after radiotherapy).
- Implant leakage or deflation of an expander implant.
- Rotation of implant (or filler port of an expander implant).

- Visible or palpable rippling of an implant.
- Thinning of overlying tissues with time.
- Chronic pain.
- Seroma and 'sloshing' of implant.
- Wound breakdown/necrosis.

In the past, concerns have been raised that systemic diseases are associated with breast implants. There is no evidence for this phenomenon, and most major manufacturers do not recommend routine replacement of implants after 5/10 years.

Outcomes

The findings of the fourth National Mastectomy and Breast Reconstruction Audit (NMBRA) are extremely useful for informing patients of likely outcomes and to compare the results of the different reconstruction options (see Further reading). Approximately 70% of immediate and 85% of delayed implant reconstruction patients are satisfied or very satisfied with the amount of rippling of their implant that can be seen or felt. Approximately 7% of implant-based reconstructions have a post-operative infection requiring removal.

Latissimus dorsi (LD) reconstruction

Basic principles

The LD reconstruction is a pedicled, autologous flap supplied by the thoracodorsal artery (see Fig. 19.1). The size of the overlying skin paddle and the amount of subcutaneous fat and muscle that is harvested will depend on the surgeon's requirements.

Types of LD reconstruction

- Extended LD flap: harvesting the maximal amount of LD muscle and fat underlying Scarpa's fascia to create a purely autologous reconstruction.
- LD and implant: the LD flap is used for coverage of an implant. This approach gives the soft feel of autologous tissue with the added volume of an implant. The implant can be totally covered by LD anteriorly or the implant pocket is created by lifting pectoralis major anteriorly and covering the lower pole with the LD flap.

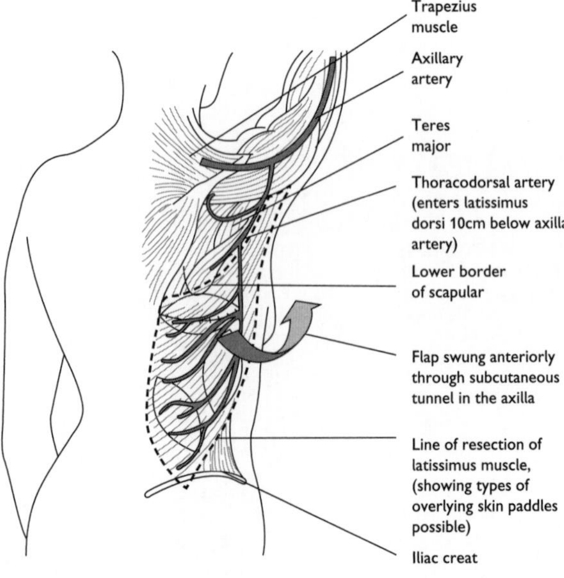

Fig. 19.1 Latissimus dorsi flap. Reproduced with permission from Chaudry MA and Winslet MC, 'The Oxford Specialist Handbook of Surgical Oncology', copyright 2009, Oxford University Press.

Advantages

- Relatively radioresistant, especially if there is no implant present.
- Good aesthetic result, even in mildly ptotic breasts.
- Use of expander implant gives adjustability.
- Robust flap with a low failure rate.
- Can be used selectively in smokers.

Disadvantages

- Removes LD function on the ipsilateral side (may affect shoulder/back/neck function).
- Donor site morbidity.
- Skin paddle is often a different colour to the chest wall skin, giving a patch appearance.
- Longer operation and recovery than implant-based reconstruction. Full recovery takes 1–3 months.
- If an implant is used, revisional surgery is likely.

Contraindications

- Previous damage to thoracodorsal pedicle.
- Active hobbies or lifestyle where weakness of LD would be a problem (e.g. sportswomen [climbers/rowers/dancers] or carers).
- Patients with pre-existing back or neck conditions.
- Severe co-morbidity—because LD flap reconstruction involves a prolonged operation and recovery.

Consent

The consent process should include discussion about the potential adverse outcomes of implant-based reconstruction if an implant is being used, as discussed in the previous section. Specifically, patients undergoing LD reconstruction should be warned about the risks of:

- Flap failure (rare).
- Donor site morbidity, including skin necrosis/breakdown and seromas.
- Chronic pain (especially from donor site).
- Weakness of back/shoulder muscles—particularly noticeable when picking up heavy bags/taking items from a high shelf/getting up out of a bath or off the floor.
- Scarring on back and around the inset skin paddle.
- Future risk of hernias (lumbar hernias).

Outcomes

See Further reading—NMBRA.

- 1.2% partial and 0.2% total flap loss.
- 9.5% risk of donor site complications (7.5% of patients require post-operative drainage of a seroma or haematoma).
- 10–15% of women are bothered by the appearance of their donor site scar.
- ~12% of women suffer shoulder or back pain most, or all, of the time following surgery.
- ~20% of women have difficulty lifting and carrying heavy objects.
- Scores for emotional, sexual, and physical well-being as well as breast appearance are higher than those of implant-based reconstruction.

Abdominal flap reconstruction

Basic principles

The abdominal flap reconstruction is an autologous flap supplied by one of the epigastric arteries (see Fig. 19.2) that can be taken as a pedicled flap or as a free flap requiring microsurgical anastomosis. Skin and subcutaneous fat are harvested from the lower abdomen, using a tranverse ellipse of resection similar to that used for an abdominoplasty procedure.

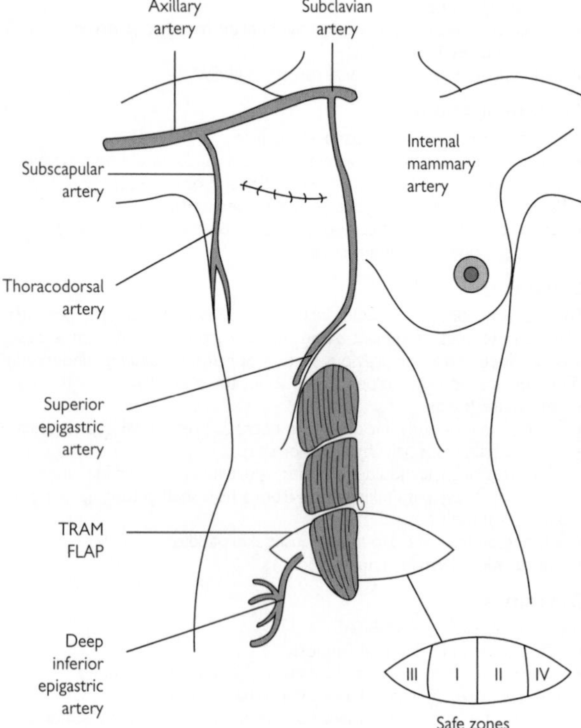

Fig. 19.2 Basic TRAM/DIEP anatomy. Safe zones I and II are the zones with the best blood supply following abdominal flap surgery. Zones III and IV often need to be sacrificed early during the operation due to their poor viability. Reproduced with permission from Chaudry MA and Winslet MC, 'The Oxford Specialist Handbook of Surgical Oncology', copyright 2009, Oxford University Press.

Types of abdominal flap reconstruction

- Pedicled TRAM (transverse rectus abdomininis muscle) flap: the viability of the skin and subcutaneous tissues is maintained by lifting the whole length of the rectus abdominis (usually on the contralateral side) based on the superior epigastric artery pedicle. The flap is then rotated and tunnelled subcutaneously to fill the breast defect.
- Free TRAM flap/muscle-sparing free TRAM flap: these are both free flaps based on the inferior epigastric artery, which runs into the rectus abdominis. Variable amounts of the rectus abdominis muscle can be preserved to maintain function.
- SIEP/DIEP flaps: these spare the abdominal muscle completely by basing the skin and fat paddle upon either the superficial (SIEP) or deep (DIEP) inferior epigastric artery. These are also free flaps requiring microsurgical anastomosis.

Advantages

- Good aesthetic result, even in ptotic or large breasts.
- A large skin paddle and tissue volume is often available.
- Rarely any need for implants.
- Robust flap with a low failure rate.
- Purely autologous tissue and, therefore, more resistant to the effects of radiotherapy than an implant-based reconstruction.
- The reconstruction ages well and often requires no revision so is a good choice for motivated young women.
- Patients get a 'tummy tuck'.

Disadvantages

- Long operation (up to 8 hours) and recovery (approximately 3 months).
- Significant donor site morbidity.
- Skin paddle is often a different colour to the chest wall skin.
- Risk of systemic complications due to the potential length of surgery.
- Large changes in the patient's weight will affect native breast differently to the reconstructed breast.
- Requires microsurgical skills to perform and requires the availability of microsurgical emergency cover out of hours.

Contraindications

- Previous abdominal surgery compromising the vascular supply (vascular contraindication).
- Significant back problems—if any of the muscle is to be harvested.
- Think carefully before performing in smokers or those with BMI over 30.
- Severe co-morbidity—because abdominal flap reconstruction involves a prolonged operation and recovery.

Consent

Specifically, patients undergoing abdominal flap reconstruction should be warned about the risks of:

- Flap failure or partial failure.
- Donor site morbidity, including skin necrosis/breakdown and seromas.
- Chronic pain (especially from donor site).

- Weakness of abdominal muscles—particularly noticeable when getting up out of a bath or off the floor.
- Abdominal scarring.
- Future risk of abdominal hernias.
- Risk of infection if a prosthetic mesh is used to strengthen or repair the abdominal musculature.
- Systemic complications, e.g. DVT/chest infection.
- Umbilical loss or stenosis.
- Risk of return to theatre in the immediate post-operative period (~12%).

Outcomes

See Further reading—NMBRA.

- 2% partial and 2% total flap loss.
- ~15% local complication rate (5% have a donor site complication).
- 75–80% of women are satisfied with their abdominal appearance.
- ~10% of women suffer abdominal bulging or tightness.
- ~5% of women have difficulty sitting up due to abdominal muscle weakness.
- Scores for emotional, sexual, and physical well-being as well as breast appearance are higher than those of implant-based reconstruction or LD-based reconstruction. Satisfaction levels are higher for free flaps than for pedicle-based flaps.

Further reading

Rainsbury D, Willett A (2012). Oncoplastic breast reconstruction—Guidelines for Best Practice ABS/BAPRAS Nov 2012. Available at: http://www.associationofbreastsurgery.org.uk/media/23851/final_oncoplastic_guidelines_for_use.pdf

Spear SL, Willey SC, Robb GL, Hammond DC, Nahabedian MY, eds (2010). *Surgery of the breast: principles and art*, 3e. Lippincott Williams & Wilkins, Philadelphia.

NMBRA. Available at: http://webarchive.nationalarchives.gov.uk/20120802111034/

http://www.ic.nhs.uk/services/national-clinical-audit-support-programme-ncasp/audit-reports/mastectomy-and-breast-reconstruction

Jones GE, ed (2010). *Bostwick's plastic and reconstructive breast surgery*, 3e. Quality Medical Publishing, St Louis.

Chapter 20

Lipomodelling

Overview

Lipomodelling is a fast-evolving technique that harvests subcutaneous fat, usually from the abdomen/flanks/thighs, and uses it for volume replacement in the breast. Fat is harvested using liposuction, and then the fat cells are separated from the tissue fluid/blood and oil that is also gathered during liposuction. Separation is usually achieved by centrifugation, but processes for washing the fat cells have also recently been developed. Fat for injection can also be enriched with adipose-derived regenerative cells (ADRCs), which may enhance graft take by maximizing vascularization of the graft (see Further reading).

Fat injection (lipomodelling) into the breast will only be successful if the fat is injected in small aliquots to an area with a good blood supply. Fat is injected in tunnels at different depths and angles to achieve a 3-dimensional increase in volume, avoiding the formation of 'fat lakes' which will form fat necrosis/oil cysts over time.

Lipomodelling is dependent upon a suitable donor site but, if fat can be harvested, lipomodelling allows the surgeon to contour the breast, depending on the specific needs of the patient. Lipomodelling may need to be repeated several times to reach the desired result; volume increases over 150–200mL can rarely be achieved in one session.

Indications

Common uses of lipomodelling include:

- Correction of contour deformities (e.g. lack of upper, medial fullness) after previous breast reconstruction or augmentation.
- To soften the contour at the edge of a breast implant.
- Filling of contour and volume deformities after previous breast-conserving surgery.
- As a volume adjunct to a previous reconstruction (e.g. to increase breast bulk after previous autologous reconstruction where the surgeon/patient wishes to avoid an implant).
- As a method of delayed breast reconstruction (see Further reading).
- Breast augmentation (lipomodelling in this setting will only give limited volume increase, often over several treatments).
- To provide soft tissue cover prior to breast augmentation or delayed reconstruction.

Advantages

- Liposuction of fatty areas on abdomen/flanks/thighs is usually welcome.
- Quick to perform and gives a natural autologous feel.

Disadvantages

- There is a significant learning curve to master all its applications.
- Donor site can become cosmetically unsatisfactory if fat is not evenly harvested.
- Theoretical risk of interference with mammographic screening causing an increase in recurrence rates. However, there is currently no evidence to demonstrate interference with mammographic screening or a higher risk of local recurrence with this technique.

Complications

Specifically, patients undergoing lipomodelling should be warned about the risks of:

- Fat necrosis/oil cysts and, therefore, increased risk of diagnostic biopsy after their next mammographic screening to ensure all mammographic changes are benign. Possible risk of cancer recurrence.
- Donor site morbidity, including bruising, infection, visceral injury, and lumpiness.
- Lipomodelling often needs repeating until the desired cosmetic result is achieved.

Further reading

Lipomodelling guidelines for breast surgery Joint guidelines from the Association of Breast Surgery, the British Association of Plastic, Reconstructive and Aesthetic Surgeons and the British Association of Aesthetic Plastic Surgeons. Available at: http://www.bapras.org.uk/download-doc.asp?id=666

Breast reconstruction using lipomodelling after breast cancer treatment (IPG417). Available at: http://guidance.nice.org.uk/ipg417

Perez-Cano R, Vranckx, J, Lasso J, *et al.* (2012). Prospective trial of adipose-derived regenerative cell (ADRC)—enriched fat grafting for partial mastectomy defects: the RESTORE-2 trial. *Eur J Surg Oncol* **38**, 382–9.

Rainsbury D, Willett A (2012). Oncoplastic breast reconstruction—Guidelines for Best Practice ABS/BAPRAS Nov 2012. Available at: http://www.associationofbreastsurgery.org.uk/media/23851/final_oncoplastic_guidelines_for_use.pdf

Spear SL, Willey SC, Robb GL, Hammond DC, Nahabedian MY, eds (2010). *Surgery of the breast: principles and art*, 3e. Lippincott Williams & Wilkins, Philadelphia.

Chapter 21

Nipple-areola reconstruction

Overview

The common situations in which the need for nipple-areola reconstruction is encountered are:

- Following immediate/delayed flap reconstruction.
- After central wide local excision.
- Nipple loss following duct surgery or mastopexy/breast reduction.

General principles

Nipple reconstruction can be performed as part of a one-stage breast reconstruction. However, the final position of the nipple may change in the months following surgery, as the reconstructed breast assumes its final position. Therefore, NAC reconstruction is usually performed as a delayed procedure under local anaesthetic, 3–6 months following reconstruction.

The first stage is to re-create the nipple mound using either a local flap or a graft. This is then tattooed 3 months later to symmetrize with the contralateral NAC.

Consent and preoperative issues

Nipple reconstruction is not mandatory after breast reconstruction, and some patients decide not to bother. However, it is important to give the patient the options that are available. Before the final decision to reconstruct, it may be helpful to give the patient an artificial nipple, which can be custom-made so that the patient has some idea of the visual benefit. It can also be helpful in final positioning if reconstruction is undertaken because, if worn regularly in the lead up to surgery, the artificial nipple leaves a mark which makes positioning much more accurate. If reconstruction is undertaken, the patient should be made aware of the following possible complications:

- Loss of nipple projection, requiring revision.
- Nipple necrosis and infection.
- Asymmetry (especially if performed as a one-stage procedure).
- Donor site morbidity (if graft is used).
- Poor scarring.
- Loss of tattoo pigment.

The patient needs to be warned that, because reconstructed nipples nearly always shrink, it is often wise to make them a little too large to allow for this atrophy. Beware also that much of the 'new' nipple is made of subcutaneous fat so that a very thin patient with prominent nipples may prove difficult to match, particularly if an implant reconstruction has taken place, as the tissues may be very thin after expansion. Therefore, it is important, as in all reconstructions, to match the patient to the technique.

Marking up

The patient should be marked in the upright position prior to surgery. The position of the new NAC should be marked to achieve close symmetry with the contralateral side and should ideally be positioned on the site of maximum projection of the breast.

Nipple position can either be determined using contralateral measurements of NAC distance from the sternal notch, midline, and infra-mammary fold, or an adhesive sticker, such as an ECG dot, may be used. When marking the areola, a template of the contralateral side should be traced.

Techniques

Local flaps

Local flaps are designed to harvest skin and underlying fat in order to create a nipple mound. When designing a flap, pre-existing scars should be avoided, as this may compromise the blood supply. The general principle is to aim to produce a mound with double the height of the opposite nipple, as it will invariably lose projection with time.

Local flaps should not be closed under tension, as this leads to poor scarring, which is difficult to camouflage by tattooing, and to flattening of the mound. If necessary, a full-thickness skin graft can be used to aid closure.

If the flap site overlies an implant-based reconstruction, there may be a lack of subcutaneous tissue to create projection. A strip of underlying muscle may be raised with the skin or a filler, such as acellular dermal matrix, used. Beware of damaging the underlying prosthesis.

There are many different techniques and modifications described using locally designed flaps. The most common are described in the following bullet points. C-V flap is the most commonly used; other methods of local flap are very similar in principle to this. Following reconstruction, the site should be covered with a non-adherent dressing, which avoids direct pressure on the reconstructed mound.

C-V flap (see Fig. 21.1):

- Raise flap based on modified star design.
- Include subcutaneous fat deep to central flap.
- Wrap lateral wings around—one inferior and one superior.
- Central flap placed on top to create plateau.
- Close skin defects directly.

Skate flap (see Further reading):

- Raise flap based on semicircular design.
- Include subcutaneous fat deep to central flap.
- Close deep tissue defect to create base for nipple.
- Lateral wings are opposed to create conical projection.
- Skin defect is closed directly.

Star flap (see Further reading):

- Raise flap based on triangular design.
- Include subcutaneous fat deep to central flap.
- Oppose tips of all triangles to create mound.
- Close skin defects directly.

A major advantage of these flaps is that for, the most part, they can be done under local anaesthesia as a day case/outpatient.

Grafts

Full-thickness skin grafts can be taken from various donor sites, including the pigmented inner thigh/labia. However, due to potential donor site morbidity, the need for general anaesthetic, and morbidity at the donor site, these techniques have largely been superseded by local flaps and tattooing. Redundant breast skin (e.g. as part of a Wise pattern breast procedure) can be used as a full thickness Wolfe graft to recreate an areola, avoiding the need for tattooing.

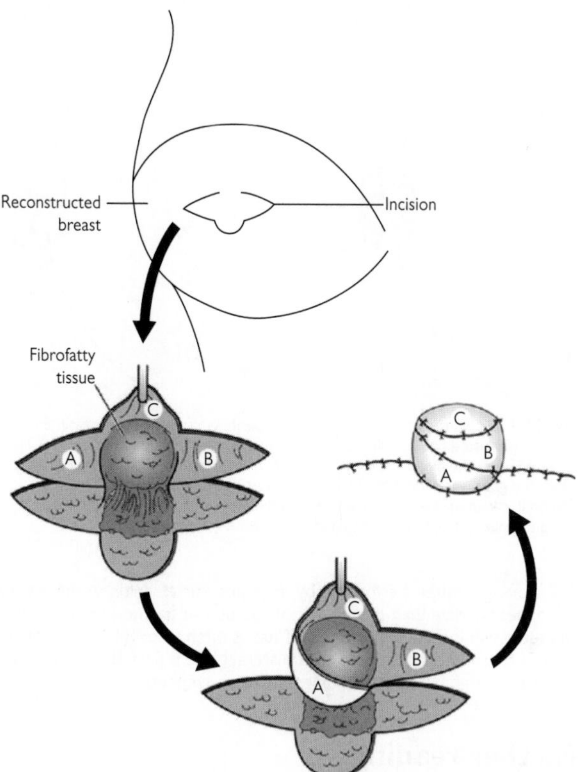

Fig. 21.1 Nipple reconstruction with a C-V flap. Reproduced with permission from Chaudry MA and Winslet MC, 'The Oxford Specialist Handbook of Surgical Oncology', copyright 2009, Oxford University Press.

If the contralateral nipple is a generous size, a free nipple graft may be harvested and placed on a de-epithelialized dermal bed (see Fig. 21.2). The two main techniques are to excise a distal wedge of the nipple, closed with a purse string suture, or to take the inferior half of the nipple (preferred) which is closed directly. This is very useful where there is a disparity between nipple size and subcutaneous fat.

Tattooing

This should be performed under local anaesthetic, at least 2 months following nipple reconstruction. The goal is to match the size, shape, and colour of the contralateral NAC. This can be done by creating a template of the opposite nipple shape and by careful matching of pigment colours.

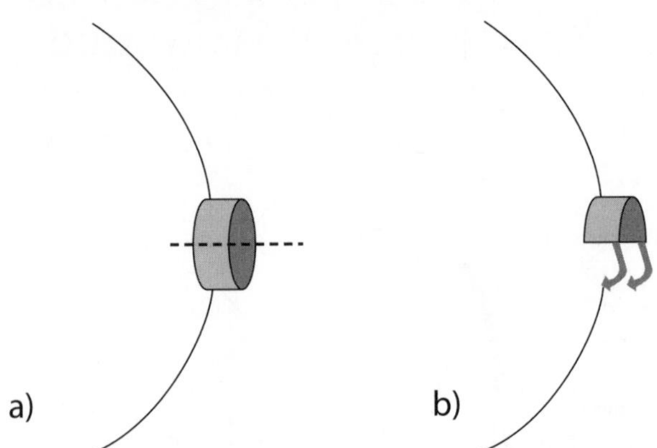

Fig. 21.2 Nipple reconstruction with a composite graft. a) The contralateral nipple is harvested by removing the inferior half of the nipple, full-thickness. b) The lower edges of the nipple are sutured to the inferior edge of the raw area from which the graft was harvested. This leaves a surprisingly normal-shaped nipple. The graft is kept in saline and is sutured on the preferred site of the new nipple by de-epithelializing the recipient site and suturing the graft down.

Tattooing is often performed by specialist nurses. Initially, the tattoo will appear darker than the desired shade due to haemosiderin, but this will settle within a couple of weeks. Tattoos often fade with time and may require repeat attempts. If the contralateral NAC is pale, the patient may wish to undergo bilateral tattooing to achieve symmetry.

Further reading

Jones GE, ed (2010). *Bostwick's plastic and reconstructive breast surgery*, 3e. Quality Medical Publishing, St Louis.

Spear SL, Willey SC, Robb GL, Hammond DC, Nahabedian MY, eds (2010). *Surgery of the breast: principles and art*, 3e. Lippincott Williams & Wilkins, Philadelphia.

Chapter 22

Breast augmentation and symmetrization surgery

Breast augmentation

Basic principles

Hypomastia may occur as a developmental or involutional process. Developmental hypomastia can be unilateral or bilateral, or secondary to a chest wall deformity. Hypomastia often results from breast involution in post-partum women; this is exacerbated by breastfeeding and significant weight loss. Inadequate breast volume can lead to a negative body image, which may affect a patient's quality of life.

Breast implant choice

Breast implant manufacture is constantly evolving and improving. The major types of breast implant are:

Silicone implants

Silicone is made up of polymeric chains; the physical properties of the silicone depend on both the chain length and the level of cross-linking between the polymers. Increased cross-linking and longer chain length results in higher viscosity and a formed stable gel (it maintains its shape when sitting or lying). Modern implants are made up of two core parts:

- Shell: tough silicone shell with a textured surface; the textured surface allows tissue adherence and ingrowth. The textured surface reduces implant movement/rotation in its pocket and capsule formation.
- Filling: cohesive gels are solid, even when cut with a knife; this results in less gel bleeding through the implant shell and less silicone leakage should an implant shell fail. The cohesiveness of the gel will determine the feel of the implant from soft through to firm.

Shape: implants are manufactured in a huge variety of sizes and in two main shapes—anatomical or round.

- Round: round implants vary in base width and in projection. The majority of breast augmentations have been performed with round implants. They eliminate the risk of implant rotation present with anatomical implants and are easier to insert. Round implants are particularly good for women who want visible enhancement to the medial cleavage area.
- Anatomical: anatomical implants provide a more naturally shaped breast implant that is fuller in the lower pole than the upper pole. Surgeons can choose an implant based upon its base width, height, and projection.

Saline implants

Widely used in the US because silicone implants were banned by the FDA during a period when it was thought that these implants caused autoimmune disease. Saline implants, if underfilled, tend to ripple and, if overfilled, result in very firm implants. Used for transumbilical breast augmentation.

Polyurethane

Polyurethane-covered implants gain very good tissue adherence and are increasingly being used for revision augmentations, particularly when rotation of an implant caused the need for revisional surgery. These implants have a polyurethane shell covering a conventional silicone implant. The polyurethane coating has a tendency to decrease capsule formation but may also delaminate from the underlying implant over time. Little data are available on the long-term outcomes of modern-generation polyurethane implants (see Further reading).

Expanders

Breast tissue expanders are made up of a silicone shell and are expanded serially in their tissue pocket using saline. Expanders are temporary implants used to create a pocket where tissues are tight and need stretching over time. The devices can be round or anatomical and can have an integrated port (e.g. Allergan 133 or Mentor Contour profile) or a filler port that is sited subcutaneously, remote from the device. Expander implants (e.g. Allergan 150 range or Mentor 'Becker' devices) combine some silicone fill (for improved contour and feel) with the flexibility of saline expansion. Expander implants are designed as permanent implants not requiring exchange.

Incision choice

- Inframammary: the most commonly used incision, as it gives the surgeon excellent views and control over pocket formation and is suitable for both subglandular and subpectoral positioning. One disadvantage is that, in patients with a short nipple-to-inframammary fold (IMF) distance, it can be difficult to site the incision in what will be the final IMF position (i.e. the scar has a tendency to ride up onto the lower breast).
- Transaxillary: the transaxillary approach has the obvious advantage of avoiding visible scars on the breast. It is used for submuscular implant placement, but the incision site does make the surgery more technically demanding. The implant pocket is either dissected bluntly using a dissector (increased risk of bleeding) or more accurately using endoscopic instruments or lighted retractors. This technique gives good control of the final IMF position.
- Periareolar: this allows for an inconspicuous scar and good access to the implant pocket through an inferior peri-areolar incision. It is an excellent option for augmentation in women with small tuberous breasts, as it flattens the breast shape, releases the lower pole constriction associated with tuberous breasts, and eliminates any areolar herniation. It is also useful when the IMF needs lowering. However, peri-areolar incisions may decrease nipple sensation, and cutting through breast ducts may result in increased bacterial contamination of the implant (which has been associated with infection and capsule formation).
- Transumbilical: this approach can be used to place saline-filled implants only; the incision does not allow sufficient access for silicone implant placement. Scarring is minimal, and little post-operative pain is reported.

Implant pocket location

Subglandular

Placement of the implant in the subglandular position will give optimal results in patients with good soft tissue coverage (subclavicular soft tissue pinch >2cm). The implant pocket is between the posterior aspect of the breast parenchyma and the anterior fascia of the pectoralis major muscle.

Subfascial

An attempt to combine the benefits of subglandular and submuscular techniques. The implant is placed under the anterior pectoralis fascia which may result in less visible implant edges, rippling, and contracture than subglandular placement. Not widely used.

Submuscular

Retropectoral placement increases soft tissue coverage over the implant, giving a more natural feel, and reduces medial visibility and rippling of the prosthesis. Disadvantages include increased post-operative pain, reduction of pectoralis major function, and 'animation' (visible lateral movement) of the implant when pectoralis major contracts.

Complications of breast augmentation

- Capsule formation: has a reported incidence of 1–30% (see Table 22.1).
- Scars at site of insertion.
- Bleeding.
- Reduced nipple/breast sensation.
- Infection: which may result in explantation of the device.
- Interference with mammographic screening: silicone devices are extremely dense on mammography and may mask some of the breast parenchyma.
- Unsatisfactory cosmetic result: outcome is very dependent on managing the patient's expectations and ensuring thorough patient education and open discussion throughout the consultation process.
- Risk of revisional surgery in the future: either due to implant failure or a change in the patient's tissues over time.
- Palpability of the implant and rippling.
- Implant rotation: occurs in 72% of anatomical breast implant augmentations.
- Leakage: silicone gel implants only leak when the shell has failed. Expanders may deflate due to a leak from the injection port site.

Tissue planning process

See Further reading. Planning a breast augmentation must allow for both the patient's wishes and also the tissue characteristics. Planning a breast augmentation should take account of the following five factors:

- Implant coverage/pocket planning.
- Implant size/volume.
- Implant type.
- Inframammary fold position.
- Incision.

This planning process must be conducted with the patient and can be further enhanced using visual aids (photos, image capture and computer planning technology, device catalogues, demonstrating a range of prostheses, interactive digital education) to try to exhibit a likely outcome range.

Table 22.1 Baker classification of capsular firmness in augmented breasts

Grade of capsule formation	Clinical signs
I	Soft breast, with no palpable implant
II (minimal firmness)	Soft breast; the implant can be palpated but is not visible.
III (moderate firmness)	The implant can be palpated easily, and distortion is visible.
IV (severe contracture)	The breast is hard and tender, with marked distortion.

Reproduced with permission from 'Classification of capsular contracture after prosthetic breast reconstruction', Spear SL, Baker JL Jr., Plast Reconstr Surg. 1995 Oct;96(5):1119-23; discussion 1124.

Beware—cases requiring specialist expertise

- Previous breast reduction or mastopexy.
- Secondary augmentation procedures.
- Chest wall deformities.
- Differential breast augmentation (non-symmetrical breasts requiring a personalized operation for each side).

Post-operative care

Drains can be used to remove any blood from the implant pocket in the first 24 hours after surgery. Careful haemostasis is key to breast augmentation, as the presence of blood in the implant pocket may contribute to capsule formation. Many surgeons use pressure garments or taping of the breasts for several weeks in the post-operative period to minimize implant movement and lateral drift of the implants.

Symmetrization surgery

Basic principles

Surgery, including breast conservation surgery, mastectomy, and mastectomy with immediate reconstruction, can leave women with significant size and shape discrepancies between their two breasts. Managing this mismatch is challenging. During the consent process for any breast surgery, women must be shown any pre-existing differences between the breasts and warned that there will be a difference following treatment, the extent of which is difficult to predict.

Options for managing asymmetry

- Reassurance and a frank discussion: reassurance that this is normal. Many women, once they have explored all possible surgical options, will opt for no further surgical symmetrization surgery. This involves the lowest level of risk to the patient and her current aesthetic appearance. Many patients do not want to have surgery or scars on their unaffected and 'normal' breast.
- Volume deficit: volume can be enhanced with breast augmentation or lipomodelling (see Chapter 20).
- Volume too large: breast reduction or liposuction.
- Ptosis: often a problem after contralateral implant-based reconstruction. Mastopexy, or breast reduction, is mainstay of treatment.

Timing of symmetrization surgery

When to perform symmetrization surgery is a personal decision. Generally, it is performed either at the time of the index procedure (more challenging) or once the ipsilateral breast has completed treatment and its size and shape have matured. Factors which influence decision-making include:

- Patient preference.
- Macromastia: patients with macromastia who are having a large reduction in volume on one side will be lopsided if the contralateral breast is not also reduced at the same time.
- Radiotherapy: radiotherapy has a relatively unpredictable effect upon final breast volume and size. Performing synchronous bilateral surgery may leave patients with asymmetry once radiotherapy is complete.
- Adjuvant chemo-/radiotherapy: patients at high risk of systemic disease should not have their adjuvant chemotherapy delayed by cosmetic contralateral surgery. Complications from contralateral surgery are common and can delay the start of adjuvant treatments.
- Theatre capacity and the availability of a skilled surgeon to work synchronously on the contralateral breast.

Further reading

de la Pena-Salcedo J, Soto-Miranda M, Lopez-Salguero J (2012). Back to the future: a 15 year experience with polyurethane foam-covered implants using the partial subfascial technique. *Aesthetic Plast Surg* **36**, 331–8.

Pompei S, Arelli F, Labardi, L, *et al.* (2001). Breast reconstruction with polyurethane implants: preliminary report. *Eur J Plast Surg* Epub 21 June 2011.

Spear SL, Willey SC, Robb GL, Hammond DC, Nahabedian MY, eds (2010). *Surgery of the breast: principles and art*, 3e. Lippincott Williams & Wilkins, Philadelphia.

Tebbetts JB, Adams WP (2005). Five critical decisions in breast augmentation. Using five measurements in 5 minutes: the high five decision support process. *Plast Reconstr Surg* **116**, 2005–16.

Jones GE, ed (2010). *Bostwick's plastic and reconstructive breast surgery*, 3e. Quality Medical Publishing, St Louis.

Further reading

Chapter 23

Recurrent breast cancer

Overview

Following initial treatment for breast cancer, the risk of recurrence is the event that patients most dread. As a consequence, minor symptoms, even if they are of no significance, can cause great anxiety. It is important, therefore, that symptoms suspicious of a recurrence are promptly investigated, so either the patient can be reassured or treatment initiated without undue delay.

Recurrences can be:

- Local: either in a conserved breast or on the chest wall following mastectomy.
- Locoregional: usually in the local draining lymph nodes of the axilla or supraclavicular fossae.
- Systemic: arising at sites distant to the breast, the most common being bone, lungs, liver, and brain.

Although these are the common sites, breast recurrences can occur almost anywhere anatomically, including as an isolated skin metastasis.

It is also important to realize that local recurrence can be associated with another asymptomatic systemic recurrence. Therefore, when a recurrence is diagnosed, it is important to make a general staging assessment of the extent of disease before the MDT formulates a treatment plan, which may involve treating both local and systemic recurrence. Management is very much a multidisciplinary activity.

Management of recurrence

Management of recurrence

Local recurrence following breast conservation

This will either be found as a lump on clinical exam or, more commonly, on mammography at follow-up. When this follows wide local excision for invasive cancer, the only option is mastectomy. This is because if the patient has already had radiotherapy, it cannot be repeated, and the recurrence suggests that the disease is more extensive than appeared initially and is radioresistant; therefore, anything less runs the risk of another recurrence at some point in the future. The possible exception to this is when a patient, for some reason, has not had previous radiotherapy. In these circumstances, if a patient was unwilling to consider mastectomy, further wide local excision could be considered, this time combined with radiotherapy; these situations will be rare though.

Local recurrence following mastectomy

This can vary in extent, from a single small nodule in a scar to a 'field change' with multiple nodules of widespread recurrence throughout the skin flaps. If radiotherapy had not been used originally, most cases will require a course of radiotherapy to the chest wall. In addition, there may be a case for surgical excision as well. With a very small area of localized recurrence, this may be quite straightforward. However, if the area is extensive, clearance may be difficult to achieve and might involve the use of flaps to cover the defect. A full assessment and MDT discussion should take place before embarking on any surgery.

Local nodal recurrence

These can occur despite axillary clearance. There is no single correct treatment, and every case needs individual assessment and discussion.

The options include:

- Local surgery to debulk the nodes, followed by a further course of systemic treatment, often chemotherapy.
- Systemic treatment on its own, using the nodes as a means of assessing response to treatment.
- Radiotherapy: this can have a place for nodes, particularly those difficult to access surgically in the supraclavicular fossa; however, there can be significant morbidity with lymphoedema following this, particularly if a node clearance has been performed.

Systemic recurrence

In addition to the physical symptoms produced, systemic recurrence can be a source of major psychological morbidity since it is systemic recurrence that leads to death. It is important to appreciate that its presence means that the cancer is no longer curable, and, even if this episode is controlled, it will recur at some time in the future, unless the patient dies of something else in the meantime. Nevertheless, with modern chemotherapy, biological modifiers, and hormone manipulation, significant control can be gained, and very worthwhile quality of life can be achieved. The majority of patients get a good response to treatment of both their first and second recurrences; thereafter, results become much less predictable.

The common sites for recurrence are:
- Bone.
- Liver.
- Lungs.
- Brain.

Management of the patient will involve:
- An assessment of disease extent.
- An assessment of the patient's physical state and suitability for treatment.
- A pathological assessment of the tumour; suitability for treatment with hormone therapy or biological modifiers, such as Herceptin®.
- A discussion with the patient and their relatives about treatment and what it involves.

In the past, diagnosis of recurrence has often been by imaging alone; however, there is an increasing argument that, where possible, a biopsy is obtained in order to reassess receptor status, as this may have changed since the original diagnosis.

Most recurrences will be treated by systemic therapy, the general principles of which are:
- Chemotherapy will produce a faster response than hormone manipulation.
- Hormone receptor-positive tumours may respond to a change of hormone therapy rather than automatically opting for chemotherapy.
- Hormone receptor-negative tumours will usually need a further course of chemotherapy, often with taxanes.
- Patients with Her-2-positive tumours who did not receive trastuzumab will benefit from that treatment.

Management of skeletal metastases and palliative care

The skeleton is probably the commonest site of first systemic recurrence. In the first instance, it may be the only site and often responds very well to treatment. There are important aspects to remember in managing skeletal metastases (see Further reading). A thorough radiological assessment and a low threshold for referral to an orthopaedic surgeon is important because:

- There may be long bone metastases which are in danger of producing a pathological fracture requiring stabilization.
- There may be vertebral body deposits that are in imminent danger of producing cord compression.

In addition, a proportion of patients may present with hypercalcaemia which requires emergency admission and treatment with:

- Intravenous rehydration.
- Intravenous bisphosphonates.

Outside these acute situations, management of bone metastases is usually by:

- A course of systemic treatment usually dictated by receptor status.
- Local radiotherapy to painful metastases or those in danger of fracture.
- Oral bisphosphonates.

Role of surgery and radiotherapy in systemic recurrence

Both these modalities have limited use in systemic recurrence. Surgery may be used:

- To biopsy an accessible recurrence, if necessary.
- For isolated liver and brain metastases which may be suitable for resection.
- To stabilize skeletal metastases.

Radiotherapy is primarily used in skeletal metastases, although it can be used for brain metastases as well.

Role of palliative care

Palliative care techniques are a discipline in themselves, and it would be pointless trying to cover them in this chapter (see 🕮 Oxford Handbook of Palliative Care, 2e (2009). Watson *et al.* Oxford University Press, Oxford, UK). It is important to remember that they are not applicable solely at the end of life, and palliative care teams have much to offer in helping in the physical management of problems related to recurrence. It is well worthwhile arranging for patients with recurrence to make contact with palliative care services in order to make an assessment of their likely needs, both physical and psychological.

Locally advanced breast cancer

There are two situations generally in which this occurs:

- As chest wall recurrence following previous surgery for breast cancer.
- As initial late presentation of primary disease.

In this latter case, it may well be associated with systemic disease so that, in this situation, a full screen for systemic disease is important. It is also important to realize that these patients may only present because their family are distressed by the smell of a necrotic fungating tumour that the patient has been hiding for some time and may have resulted in them being socially isolated. Apart from considerations of tumour treatment, they often need the care of specialist wound care services to gain control of anaerobic infection, which makes the situation even more distressing.

There is no single correct management of the local problem, and it is often harder to deal with if it is recurrence after treatment rather than initial presentation. The general approach is to:

- Use systemic therapy to reduce tumour burden.
- Following a good response, embark on salvage surgery to debulk the local disease and optimize local control.
- Use radiotherapy to consolidate control following surgery.

In some patients, even after systemic therapy, surgery is not possible, and, in these circumstances, radiotherapy, if it has not already been used, may be helpful.

Unfortunately, there is a small group of patients in whom neither physical nor pharmacological manipulation proves effective, and they need the help of both the wound care and palliative care services.

Further reading

Breast cancer (early and locally advanced). Available at: http://www.nice.org.uk/CG80.
Breast cancer (advanced). Available at: http://www.nice.org.uk/CG81.
British Association of Surgical Oncology Guidelines (1999). The management of metastatic bone disease in the United Kingdom. *Eur J Surg Oncol* **25**, 3–23. Also available at: http://www.associationofbreastsurgery.org.uk/media/4505/the_management_of_metastatic_bone_disease_in_the_united_kingdom.pdf.

Chapter 24

Management of the high-risk patient

Overview

Breast cancer is common in the population, affecting approximately one in every nine women. It is, therefore, extremely common for women to volunteer that a family member has previously been affected by breast cancer. With the help of NICE guidance (see Further reading), it is important to stratify the level of individual risk. The majority of women can be reassured that, despite their family history, they are not at an increased risk of breast cancer. Those with a significant family history should be offered appropriate early screening and genetic assessment, if applicable.

Genetic mutations

Breast cancer mutations can be:

- Somatic (non-inheritable), i.e. sporadic 90%: due to failure of DNA repair mechanism of both copies of the gene. Sporadic mutations are the most common cause of cancer. The likelihood of sporadic mutations increases with age (see Fig. 24.1).
- Germline (inheritable), 5–10%: breast cancer germline mutations demonstrate an autosomal dominant pattern, i.e. inherit one abnormal copy and one normal copy from parents. Inheritance of two abnormal copies is not compatible with life. Only when the DNA in the normal copy mutates can cancer develop. This occurs at a younger age than sporadic cancer, as only one copy of the DNA has to mutate.

It is likely there are many germline mutations which will confer a range of breast cancer risk. So far, the genetic mutations identified have a high lifetime risk (>40% and up to 80% for the BRCA genes) of cancer susceptibility (high penetrance genes).

- The breast cancer susceptibility genes (BRCA1 and BRCA2) are responsible for 2–5% of all breast cancers. Women carrying these genes have a 55–80% lifetime chance of developing breast cancer. If they have large enough families, these women often have three or four affected members at a young age. Also linked with ovarian, bowel, and prostate cancer. BRCA2 is associated with male breast cancer.
- Mutation in p53 (Li Fraumeni syndrome) causes early-onset breast cancer, along with brain tumours, leukaemias, childhood sarcomas, and adrenocortical carcinomas.
- Mutation in one of several mismatch repair genes is linked to breast cancer as well as bowel (hereditary non-polyposis colorectal cancer), endometrial, ovarian, pancreatic, and stomach cancers.
- Mutation in CHEK2 doubles the background risk of breast cancer and appears to be involved in many families where two cases are identified.
- Mutations in PTEN (Cowden's syndrome), STK11/LKB1 (Peutz–Jeghers), and ATM (ataxia telangiectasia) are also occasionally a cause of familial breast cancer.

However, each family needs to be assessed on its own merits, remembering that the high incidence of breast cancer (1 in 9) means that many women will have an affected relative merely by chance, rather than due to a genetic abnormality. Indeed, over 85% of women with an affected first-degree relative will never be affected themselves, and over 85% of affected individuals have no significant family history.

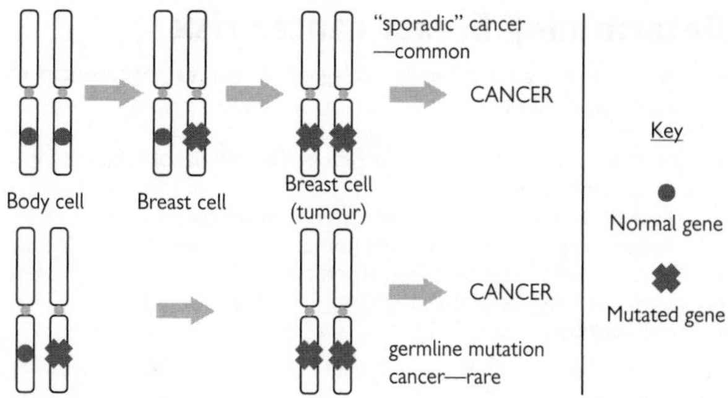

Fig. 24.1 The two-hit theory. Mutations in both copies of the genes must be present for a cancer to develop. This can occur sporadically due to chance or one mutated copy of the gene can be inherited as a germline mutation.

Determining breast cancer risk

Preliminary identification of families at higher risk comes from assessment of the patient's family history.

Need to:

- Take an accurate, extended family history. Definitions of relatives for NICE guidance are:
    - First-degree relative is mother, sister, or daughter.
    - Second-degree relative is grandmother, aunt, or niece.
- Need both sides of family: paternal and maternal.
- Confirm histology of cancer diagnoses (including ovarian).
- Age at diagnosis.

Factors that predict for likely germline mutation and increased cancer susceptibility:

- Number of breast cancer cases.
- Number of confirmed ovarian cancer cases.
- Any woman with both breast and ovarian primaries.
- Ages of diagnoses (generally, <50 is 'young').
- Any bilateral breast cancer.
- Any male breast cancer.
- Ashkenazi Jewish ancestry.

Assessment of other risk factors, including;

- Female sex.
- Increasing age.
- Oestrogen exposure: endogenous oestrogen, age at menarche and menopause, number of full-term pregnancies, and age at first pregnancy. Exogenous oestrogens, such as contraceptive hormones and HRT.
- Pathological high-risk factors, such as LCIS, ADH, multiple papillomas.
- Alcohol intake.
- Weight.

An easy way to accurately assess a patient's risk is to use 'risk assessment software', such as the IBIS risk evaluator (see Further reading). This software assesses a patient's individual risk and evaluates for age, BMI, oestrogen exposure, previous high-risk pathology (e.g. ADH), and family history. The software outputs a family tree and a 10-year and lifetime risk of breast cancer for that individual.

NICE guidance—levels of breast cancer risk

Stratifying the level of risk into one of three categories not only gives patients and clinicians knowledge of the future risk of breast cancer, but also determines what screening and future management will be offered (see Table 24.1).

High-risk: lifetime risk >30%

- Four breast cancers in family at any age; three <60; two < average age 50.
- One breast <50 (or two breast cancers <60) plus one ovarian cancer.
- Two ovarian cancers.
- One male breast cancer plus female breast cancer before 50 (or plus two breast cancers <60).

Table 24.1 Summary of the NICE guidance as to 10-year and lifetime risk of breast cancer for each risk category

Level of risk	10-year risk of breast cancer	Lifetime risk of breast cancer	Management
At or near population risk	<3%	<17%	Refer back to primary care
Raised risk	3–8%	17–30%	Managed in secondary care (breast family history clinic)
High	>8%	>30%	Refer to tertiary care for genetic assessment and testing, if appropriate

Familial breast cancer ☞ http://www.nice.org.uk/CG41.

Raised risk: lifetime risk between 17 and 30%

- One first-degree relative breast <40.
- One first- plus one second-degree relative breast cancer any age.
- Two first-degree relatives breast cancer any age.

At or near population risk: lifetime risk <17%

- Non-significant family history.

Genetic testing

At present, genetic testing on the NHS is only offered to those with a 10%, or greater, likelihood of detecting a mutation (not a 10% risk of developing breast cancer). This risk can be calculated using softwares, such as the BOADICEA, BRCAPro, or IBIS evaluator.

Without gene testing, the highest predictable risk of carrying a gene or getting breast cancer is 50%, i.e. a 1:2 chance of inheriting an abnormal gene from either mother or father. If you carry that gene, then you have a lifetime risk of breast cancer of 80%.

Note that usually testing is only offered if there is a live affected individual with cancer who can be gene-tested, however new NICE guidance now allows genetic testing on those with an affected relative who is unavailable for testing.

BRCA mutation testing is not 100% sensitive and has a significant false negative rate. A positive test means you carry the gene, but a negative test does not mean you do not carry the gene. Prior to testing, a risk estimation is made of the likelihood and counselling offered, plus other strategies, such as early screening, are discussed.

Those likely to be BRCA1/2-tested are:

- Three or more cases <60 (breast only).
- One breast case <50 and one ovarian case.
- Two ovarian cases.
- (Two breasts <50 is just on the borderline).
- Ashkenazi ancestry.

Take blood from a living, affected family member.

If a causative mutation in BRCA1/2 can be identified, then can offer predictive testing to other family members.

Management of the higher risk patient

Patients should have had their level of risk assessed. Patients at or near population risk should be reassured and discharged back to primary care. They should be advised that, if their level of risk changes (i.e. another family member is diagnosed with breast cancer), then they will need to be reassessed.

Screening

Early screening should be offered for those at raised or high risk of breast cancer. This will take the form of mammographic screening or MRI screening or both (see Table 24.2). Those with TP53 mutations are very susceptible to genetic damage caused by X-rays; these women should ONLY be offered MRI screening. Screening of high-risk women should be performed under the auspices of the NHSBSP, subject to the same QA standards (see Chapter 2).

Prior to enrolment to a breast cancer surveillance programme and at each subsequent change in the programme, women should be provided with a documented plan that includes:

- Written patient information and discussion on mammography and MRI, including the risks and benefits.
- A clear description of the methods and intervals.
- The reasons for any changes to the surveillance plan.
- Sources of support and further information (see Further reading—NICE guidance).

Risk management

Those at raised risk of breast cancer can alter their level of future risk by modifying their risk factors or by undergoing risk-reducing treatments.

Women at raised or high risk of breast cancer should be advised of their risk factors for breast cancer and of the benefits of risk modification (see Table 24.3).

Risk-reducing treatments

Risk reduction is a complex topic, and many patients are very emotive, as many have personal experience of family members being treated for breast cancer. All options for risk reduction, including surveillance only and no treatment at all, should be discussed. A specialist clinical psychologist can be invaluable to the patient to clarify their thinking and values prior to making a final decision.

Risk-reducing surgery

Risk-reducing surgery for the breast really means risk-reducing mastectomy. The amount of breast tissue removed during the mastectomy determines the level of risk reduction; the risk reduction is approximately 92–99%. Sparing the nipple inevitably leads to a better cosmetic result but also leaves ductal tissue behind the nipple; patients should be warned that this increases their level of future breast cancer by 2–5%. All patients considering risk reduction surgery should have up-to-date

Table 24.2 NICE guidance for breast screening in higher risk women

Age (years)	Mammography	MRI
20–29	Not available	Only for those at exceptionally high risk (annual risk >1%), e.g. TP53 carriers
30–39	Individualized screening should be offered for known mutation carriers	Annual MRI for those at high risk (10-year risk >8%), including those known to be mutation carriers
40–49	For women with a raised or high risk of breast cancer (10-year risk >3%)	Annual MRI for women: >20% 10-year risk of breast cancer >12% 10-year risk of breast cancer with dense breast pattern on mammography Known high-risk mutation carriers
>50	3-yearly screening under the NHSBSP Annual mammography up to age 70 for those at high risk	Not available

Familial breast cancer http://www.nice.org.uk/CG41. 1.4.4 surveillance.

Table 24.3 Risk-modifying behaviours to reduce future risk of breast cancer

Risk factor	Risk-reducing behaviour
HRT	Avoidance of HRT or keeping the treatment course as short as possible
Hormonal contraception	Advise those over age of 35 of slightly increased risk of breast cancer. BRCA carriers taking hormones have an increased risk of breast cancer but a reduction in their ovarian cancer risk
Breastfeeding	Reduces future risk of breast cancer
Alcohol	Excess alcohol consumption increases breast cancer risk but also reduces cardiovascular risk at low levels of consumption
Smoking	Stop-smoking advice
Weight and physical exercise	Women should be informed of the increased risk of breast cancer in overweight, post-menopausal women. Exercise will help reduce risk

screening radiology and have seen a clinical psychologist prior to their surgery being finalized.

Risk-reducing oophorectomy should be offered to those at high risk of ovarian cancer (BRCA carriers). The risk of ovarian cancer in BRCA carriers does not start until age 40 (BRCA 1) or 50 (BRCA 2); therefore, there is no rush to remove the ovaries prior to these ages, as the health benefits of the ovaries at a young age clearly outweigh the risks.

Following oophorectomy, a woman will be rendered post-menopausal, and this will reduce her risk of future breast cancer by 50%. This risk reduction alone may be enough, for some women, in eliminating the need for breast surgery.

Endocrine prevention

Chemoprevention of breast cancers with 5 years of tamoxifen or raloxifene is now licensed in the UK following a recent NICE consultation (see Further reading). This is only offered to moderate and high risk women. There is some evidence that tamoxifen, raloxifene, and anastrozole reduce the incidence of ER-positive breast cancers; however, there is no survival benefit (see Further reading).

Support services

All women should be given written information throughout their journey through primary, secondary, or tertiary care. This should detail their level of risk, lifestyle advice, contact information, and a summary of the discussions that have occurred. It is recommended that all patients with a family history have access to nursing support (such as a breast care nurse) and a clinical psychologist, preferably with a special interest in breast cancer. Information should also be provided on local support groups. These patients with a family history have complex problems that are best dealt with by a specialist multidisciplinary team in an environment where patients are given adequate time for discussion and contemplation.

Further reading

Familial breast cancer. Available at: http://www.nice.org.uk/CG41

NICE. Available at: http://www.nice.org.uk/CG164

Fisher B, Costantino JP, Wickerham DL, *et al.* (2005). Tamoxifen for the prevention of breast cancer: current status of the National Surgical Adjuvant Breast and Bowel Project P-1 study. *J Natl Cancer Inst* **97**, 1652–62.

Vogel V, Constantino J, Wickerham D, *et al.* (2010). Update of the National Surgical Adjuvant Breast and Bowel Project Study of Tamoxifen and Raloxifene (STAR) P-2 Trial: Preventing breast cancer. *Cancer Prev Res* **3**, 696–706.

Lostumbo L, Carbine N, Wallace J (2010). Prophylactic mastectomy for the prevention of breast cancer. *Cochrane Database Syst Rev* **10**, CD002748.

Chapter 25

Research and audit

Overview

Within the NHS, breast surgeons have made enormous national contributions to audit and research. Demonstrating a continuing involvement with audit is an important component of both appraisal and revalidation. This is particularly so for breast surgeons, as participation in NHSBSP screening audit is an important part of a screening unit's inspection process. Aside from this, in pure terms, knowledge of research methods and process is an important part of training, even if you do not carry out any research yourself. Often, the distinction between research and audit becomes blurred. One way of seeing the difference is to regard research as finding out what we should be doing and audit as seeing whether we are doing it. In other words, audit is involved with looking at the way we work and how effective it is, which forms the first part of the audit loop. In this concept, we:

- Analyse and identify problems in what we do.
- Formulate and implement strategies to correct them.
- Re-analyse the situation to see whether the expected improvements have occurred.

To audit effectively, a standard, against which to compare our performance, is required. In contrast to this, research does not necessarily need standards because this is the process whereby we extend our knowledge. The audit process may raise questions which research can be used to answer so that another way of looking at the differences between the two is to say that audit raises the questions and research attempts to answer them. To accomplish both of these activities, certain tools are needed, without which the whole process can become pointless.

Tools for research and audit

Tools for research and audit

Before embarking on either of these activities, it is important to look at several issues if whatever you do is going to be effective.

Background literature or fact search

It is important to establish what is known already. Somebody else may have answered what is a new question to you. Even if it has, you need to evaluate how they have done it and whether their methods were sound and their conclusions justified. Similarly, in audit, you need to know what standard you are judging against and whether any exist. It is often wise to let somebody completely independent look at the idea, as they will often point out things that you have forgotten. For a pure research project, it will often be impossible to go ahead without some form of external peer review.

What resources are needed?

It is almost impossible to carry out any project without resource, be it patient records, specimens, laboratory support, IT facilities, access to a good database, secretaries, or nurses. What you are going to do needs mapping out and a shopping list produced to make it work. An important component often forgotten in planning is time—you need to ask yourself 'Do I, or the others involved, have the necessary time?' Following from that is the support and goodwill needed from other people. Scientific projects may need the help of either a university or research institute.

Do I have the resources?

Very simple audit projects may need very little resource and be easily deliverable; however, as projects become complex, more is needed, and most research projects need some form of funding. This will need costing out and a decision made as to where the money is coming from.

Do I need statistical advice?

This may not be relevant for audit projects, but anything that compares outcomes in a numerical way may need statistical analysis in order to have validity. This needs to be built into the plan because it may influence the numbers of specimens, patients, or events that are needed for the work to be valid. For projects that require ethical approval, it may be impossible to obtain without submitting a statistical analysis.

Research and ethics approval

This is an extremely important aspect to consider. An audit may not require ethics approval; however, if there is doubt, advice should be taken from the appropriate ethics committee. For anything that has, what could be called, an element of research, a formal application must be made for ethical approval to the ethics committee related to the institution where the research is to be conducted. It must also be remembered that research involving patients or specimens from patients requires patient consent. For the application, details will be needed of:

- Rationale for the project.
- Methods to be employed.

- Numbers of patients or specimens required.
- Statistical basis for numbers.
- Who will be carrying out the project.
- Sample of information leaflets and consent.
- Details of how confidentiality will be maintained.

Most applications can now be completed online by accessing the research ethics website.

Research and development committee

The Research and Development department will be interested in any extra costs that may be incurred as a result of a research study. In many units, funding for research must be found before the study can begin to recruit. Close links with research and development and ethics committees are very helpful and will help to speed up what can be a very lengthy and convoluted paper process. Performing research requires long-term planning, persistence, and patience.

Disseminating information from research and audit

Having completed audit or research, you will want to communicate your results to other people. Depending on the nature of the work, a variety of forums exist:

- Local meetings.
- National meetings.
- International meetings.
- Journals.

In deciding which of these forums to use, you need to consider the group that it will be of most interest to. Is it information mainly of interest to a local audience or is it something that would be of interest nationally or even internationally? Is it primarily clinical in basis or purely scientific? Does it have broad interest within the breast community or to a specific clinical group, for instance, surgeons as opposed to radiologists? By addressing these issues, you are much more likely to succeed in presenting your work than by randomly submitting it.

Clinical trials and levels of evidence

Evidence-based medicine and management guidelines are based on levels of evidence. It is important you have some basic understanding of these (see Table 25.1).

Recommendations can subsequently be made about the direction of clinical practice, based upon the available data (see Table 25.2).

Types of clinical trials

For information on the difference between the designs of clinical trials and how to review the results of these trials, see Further reading (Young and Solomon).

The purpose of a trial is to answer specific questions about the effects of a treatment.

- Explanatory trials (phase I and II trials) evaluate the biological effects of treatment on host and tumour in small numbers of subjects to guide decisions about further research.
- Pragmatic trials (phase III and IV trials) evaluate the practical effects of treatments.

The distinction is important because treatments which have desirable biological effects (e.g. the ability to kill cancer cells and cause tumour shrinkage) may not have desirable effects in practice (i.e. may not lead to improvement in duration or quality of life). For example, many drugs with strong anti-tumour effects are so toxic that patients are unable to tolerate and derive benefit from them.

The evaluation of new cancer treatments usually involves progression through a series of clinical trials.

Phase I trials

Evaluate relationship between dose and toxicity, and aim to establish a maximum tolerable dose and schedule of administration.

Small numbers of patients are treated at successively higher doses until the maximum acceptable degree of toxicity is reached. The maximum tolerable dose is defined as the maximum dose at which dose-limiting toxicity occurs in less than one-third of patients tested. This design is based on experience rather than data and is predicated on the assumption that the maximum tolerable dose is also the most effective anticancer dose.

Phase II trials

Screen treatments for their anti-tumour effects to identify those worthy of further evaluation.

They usually include highly selected patients, excluding those with 'non-evaluable' disease, and use tumour response rate as the primary measure of outcome. Their sample size is calculated to distinguish active from inactive drugs, according to whether the response rate is greater or less than some arbitrary level, often 20%. The resulting sample size is

Table 25.1 Levels of evidence, as agreed by the Scottish Intercollegiate Guidelines Network (SIGN) (see Further reading)

1++	High-quality meta-analyses, systematic reviews of RCTs, or RCTs with a very low risk of bias
1+	Well-conducted meta-analyses, systematic reviews of RCTs, or RCTs with little risk of bias
1–	Meta-analyses, systematic reviews of RCTs, or RCTs with a high risk of bias
2++	High-quality systematic reviews of case control or cohort studies. High-quality case control or cohort studies with a very low risk of confounding or bias and a high probability that the relationship is causal
2+	Well-conducted case control or cohort studies with a low risk of confounding or bias and a moderate probability that the relationship is causal
2–	Case control or cohort studies with a high risk of confounding or bias and a significant risk that the relationship is not causal
3	Non-analytic studies, e.g. case reports, case series
4	Expert opinion

http://www.sign.ac.uk/guidelines/fulltext/50/annexb.html.

Table 25.2 SIGN grades of recommendation, based upon the levels of available evidence

Grade of recommendation	Recommendation
A	At least one meta-analysis, systematic review, or RCT rated as 1++ and directly applicable to the target population; *or* A body of evidence consisting principally of studies rated as 1+, directly applicable to the target population and demonstrating overall consistency of results
B	A body of evidence, including studies rated as 2++, directly applicable to the target population and demonstrating overall consistency of results; *or* Extrapolated evidence from studies rated as 1++ or 1+
C	A body of evidence, including studies rated as 2+, directly applicable to the target population and demonstrating overall consistency of results; *or* Extrapolated evidence from studies rated as 2++
D	Evidence level 3 or 4; *or* Extrapolated evidence from studies rated as 2+

http://www.sign.ac.uk/guidelines/fulltext/50/annexb.html.

inadequate to provide a precise estimate of activity. For example, a phase II trial with 24 patients and an observed response rate of 33% has a 95% confidence interval of 16–55%. While tumour response rate is a reasonable endpoint for assessing the anticancer activity of a drug, it is not an adequate surrogate for patient benefit.

Phase II trials are suitable for guiding decisions about further research but are not suitable for making or guiding decisions about patient management. However, the literature is often confusing because phase II trials are often reported and interpreted as if they do provide answers to questions about patient management

Phase III trials

Determine the usefulness of treatments in patient management.

Questions about patient management tend to be comparative since they involve choices between alternatives, i.e. an experimental vs the current standard management. The current standard may include other anticancer treatments or may be the best supportive care without specific anticancer therapy. The aim of a phase III trial is to estimate the difference in outcomes associated with a difference in treatments, sometimes referred to as the treatment effect.

Ideally, alternative treatments are compared by administering them to groups of patients which are equivalent in all other respects. Randomized controlled phase III trials are the best, and often only reliable, means of determining the usefulness of treatments in patient management.

Phase IV

Monitor the effects of treatments which have been incorporated into clinical practice.

Setting up clinical trials and studies

Clinical trials and studies are probably the commonest research activity that clinicians working in breast units become involved with. The trials and studies can involve all modalities of therapy, surgery, radiotherapy, and medical oncology as well as related clinical areas. Clinical trials are very carefully regulated; many relating to breast cancer are run by national organizations or groups, rather than being purely drug company-sponsored, and frequently involve multiple centres. The trial protocol will often have received multicentre ethical approval (MREC), but it is still necessary for it to be put before the hospitals local ethical committee (LREC). In order for it to get through this process, it will be necessary to have:

- A local principle investigator.
- Adequate resource to run the trial.
- Sufficient numbers of whatever group of patients are being studied.

Integrated software (IRAS) is now universally available which streamlines the application process in an online format (see Further reading). Modern trials and studies require a very significant amount of documentation, which must be carefully recorded. This begins with the consenting process for entering patients into studies and continues throughout the course of the study. Often, the whole process is helped by having trial nurses, who can help with much of the routine day-to-day organization.

It is now expected that those involved with trials, both in organization and entering patients, will have attended a course on Good Clinical Practice in relation to trials. Failure to have attended such a course may well prevent someone from becoming the principle investigator for a trial locally.

Conclusion

Research and audit can seem daunting but can be made easier if you:
- Are well organized.
- Ask for help.
- Do background work thoroughly.

Further reading

Young J, Solomon, M (2009). How to critically appraise an article. *Nat Clin Pract Gastroenterol Hepatol* **6**, 82–91.
SIGN Guidelines. Available at: http://www.sign.ac.uk/guidelines/fulltext/50/annexb.html.
IRAS Integrated Research Application System. Available at: http://www.myresearchproject.org.uk.

Chapter 26

Complaints, mistakes, and how to minimize problems

Overview

In a high-profile specialty where the patient and family are understandably anxious, it is inevitable that, for whatever reason, the interaction between the surgeon and the patient may occasionally not work well. In addition, other members of the team, or the wider institution, may not fulfill the patient's expectations.

The consequence is a complaint. If the complaint is not handled well, the consequence is litigation.

Principles of dealing with a complaint:

- Take all complaints seriously; they often have some basis.
- If a complaint is made, it may just be the tip of an iceberg problem.
- Respond rapidly to complaints; do not let them fester.
- Be prepared to swiftly offer an interview and an apology.
- There will be local guidelines, so stick to them and ensure all documentation, including responses, are properly filed.
- Complaints often represent a failure of team working. There should be regular meetings of the Breast Unit when complaints can be discussed in a non-judgemental manner.
- Complaints represent an opportunity to make things better for the patient and thus should be welcomed. So often, patients just want an explanation and an apology. Therefore, acknowledge errors; apologize, and respond rapidly.

How to prevent incidents

Never forget lawyers deal in paper. In civil law, the basis of proof is based on the balance of probability. This means that, if, on the evidence, the judge feels that it is 50.1% likely that something untoward happened as a result of an action, that action will be deemed negligent. Write clear handwritten or computer-generated notes, which are signed, timed, and dated.

- Poor notes = poor defence.
- No notes = no defence.

Delay in the diagnosis of breast cancer is the most frequent cause of litigation in breast disease.

Partly, this is because the most difficult decision in an outpatient breast clinic is to decide whether the patient has a discrete lump or whether the area of concern is merely an area of vague nodularity.

Therefore, what you write and, in particular, draw is of crucial importance when litigation starts 4 years later.

For example, consider the following scenario where the drawing of the breast and the area is labelled 'Lump'. Most experts and lawyers will believe that the surgeon found a lump. The situation is exacerbated if the clinician then fills it in to make it look solid. Most patients in a breast clinic do not have a lump, so do not draw one. Patients have vague indeterminate areas of nodularity about which they are concerned. So try to be accurate:

Write 'Area of concern to the patient. No discrete lump.'

The issue in delay in diagnosis litigation is 'did the surgeon believe the patient had a lump or not?' If the word lump is written, experts and lawyers will believe there was a lump and will want to know why it was not properly investigated or discussed.

All breast experts are familiar with the patient who thinks she has a lump but, in fact, has a vaguely nodular/lumpy area. It is a common presentation.

Expectations of how a vaguely nodular area is investigated and not followed up are different from where the word lump has been written.

Where are you vulnerable?

Poorly organized or staffed clinics

A diagnostic breast clinic involves clinical examination, probable mammography, and an U/S plus a smaller number of new patients having a core biopsy or cyst aspiration.

Thus, the lack of a breast radiologist or too many patients for that breast radiologist will result in delays in processing patients, overcrowded waiting rooms, and complaints.

Doctors and managers must work together to ensure a smooth and seamless experience for the patient. Retail is detail. Think how much you appreciate interminable waits and wearing backless gowns, and recognize that these sorts of indignities start to irritate already anxious patients.

Is it a lump?

As already noted, you must state clearly whether that patient has a lump or non-specific nodularity in the area of concern to the patient.

The pregnant breast

Many pregnant women develop concerns about possible sinister changes.

The availability of good-quality contemporary U/S of the breast has done much to improve our ability to reassure this group of patients, and there should be no hesitation to use U/S. Such patients should be offered rapid, if not open, access to a diagnostic breast clinic if they have continuing concerns during their pregnancy.

Sometimes, the cause is a fibroadenoma. It is usually possible to reassure the patient and to then offer a clinical and an U/S review when they have delivered and finished breastfeeding.

Implants

Less of a problem these days, as breast MRI is much more available. Occasionally, a non-specialist breast radiologist may baulk at doing a core biopsy for fear of damaging the implant. If this is the case, it is in the patient's best interests for her to be referred to a breast radiologist who does have these skills. These patients must be discussed at an MDM.

Failure of multidisciplinary working

The failure for key members of the MDT to communicate effectively and work cohesively is a frequent cause of a delay in diagnosis. MDTs must have adequate clerical and administrative support.

Oncoplastic surgery

It is vital that the patient has a realistic expectation of what can be achieved together with the risks. Decisions and advice should be carefully documented. It is good practice to copy clinic letters to the patient.

Decision-making in oncoplastic surgery may well require two, or more, clinic visits. A list of all the complications related to a particular procedure must be written down as they are discussed with the patient.

Clinical photographs are an important part of oncoplastic surgery. Patients must have an opportunity to see photographs of both good and bad results (see Further reading—ABS oncoplastic guidelines).

The grid

It is helpful to structure a diagnostic triple assessment by using the following grid.

In breast disease, each modality is marked from 1 to 5. Thus, B2 = benign core biopsy and M5 = mammogram reveals malignancy.

Thus, set a grid (see Table 26.1).

- Each score should be circled.
- If the scores are all 5, e.g. P5, M5, U5, B5, then, after discussion in the MDM, the patient can confidently be diagnosed as having breast cancer.
- If all the scores circled are 2, e.g. P2, M2, U2, B2, then the patient has a benign problem.
- Beware the discordant triple assessment.
- A pattern of results, such as P3, M4, U3, B1, is discordant, and it is essential that the reasons for this discordance are discussed at an MDM, and an agreed plan to resolve this discordance must be agreed.

Table 26.1 A grid is useful for demonstrating concordance between the different elements of assessment.

	Abbreviation	**1 Normal**	**2 Benign**	**3 Uncertain**	**4 Suspicious**	**5 Cancer**
Clinical/ palpable	P	1	2	3	4	5
Mammogram	M	1	2	3	4	5
Ultrasound	U	1	2	3	4	5
Biopsy	B	1	2	3	4	5

Circle the appropriate number for each element of the assessment. Non-concordance should promote multidisciplinary discussion and reassessment.

Index

C

D

T

U